O   R   L

OXFORD RHEUMATOLOGY LIBRARY

Systemic Lupus Erythematosus

BMA

BMA Library

British Medical Association
BMA House
Tavistock Square
London
WC1H 9JP

Tel: 020 7383 6625
Email: bma-library@bma.org.uk
Web: bma.org.uk/library

Location: _WD 380_

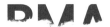

ORL

OXFORD RHEUMATOLOGY LIBRARY

Systemic Lupus Erythematosus

Edited by

Professor Caroline Gordon

Professor of Rheumatology, College of Medical and Dental Sciences,
University of Birmingham, UK

Professor David Isenberg

Diamond Jubilee Arthritis Research UK Professor of Rheumatology,
University College London, London, UK

OXFORD
UNIVERSITY PRESS

OXFORD
UNIVERSITY PRESS

Great Clarendon Street, Oxford, OX2 6DP,
United Kingdom

Oxford University Press is a department of the University of Oxford.
It furthers the University's objective of excellence in research, scholarship,
and education by publishing worldwide. Oxford is a registered trade mark of
Oxford University Press in the UK and in certain other countries

First Edition published in 2016

Impression: 1

Published in the United States of America by Oxford University Press
198 Madison Avenue, New York, NY 10016, United States of America

British Library Cataloguing in Publication Data

Data available

Library of Congress Control Number: 2015951530

ISBN 978–0–19–873918–0

Printed in Great Britain by
Clays Ltd, St Ives plc

Oxford University Press makes no representation, express or implied, that the
drug dosages in this book are correct. Readers must therefore always check
the product information and clinical procedures with the most up-to-date
published product information and data sheets provided by the manufacturers
and the most recent codes of conduct and safety regulations. The authors and
the publishers do not accept responsibility or legal liability for any errors in the
text or for the misuse or misapplication of material in this work. Except where
otherwise stated, drug dosages and recommendations are for the non-pregnant
adult who is not breast-feeding

Links to third party websites are provided by Oxford in good faith and
for information only. Oxford disclaims any responsibility for the materials
contained in any third party website referenced in this work.

Contents

v

Contributors

Dr Graciela S. Alarcón

Division of Clinical Immunology and Rheumatology, University of Alabama at Birmingham, AL, USA

Dr Nicola Ambrose

Adolescent and Adult Rheumatology Unit, University College London Hospitals, London, UK

Dr Sarah Doaty

University of California Los Angeles, Los Angeles, CA, USA

Professor Caroline Gordon

College of Medical and Dental Sciences, University of Birmingham, UK

Professor Bevra H. Hahn

University of California Los Angeles, Los Angeles, CA, USA

Dr Yiannis Ioannou

Adolescent and Adult Rheumatology Unit, University College London Hospitals, London, UK

Dr Anthony Isaacs

Centre for Rheumatology, University College Hospital, London, UK

Professor David Isenberg

Centre for Rheumatology, University College London, London, UK

Dr April Jorge

Northwestern University Feinberg School of Medicine, Chicago, IL, USA

Dr S. Sam Lim

Department of Medicine, Division of Rheumatology, Emory University, Atlanta, GA, USA

Dr Peter Lloyd

University of California Los Angeles, Los Angeles, CA, USA

Dr Maria Mouyis

Centre for Rheumatology, University College Hospital, London, UK

Dr Claire Louise Murphy

Adolescent and Adult Rheumatology Unit, University College London Hospitals, London, UK

Professor Anisur Rahman

Centre for Rheumatology, University College London, London, UK

Professor Rosalind Ramsey-Goldman

Northwestern University Feinberg School of Medicine, Chicago, IL, USA

Dr Ben Rhodes

Department of Rheumatology, Queen Elizabeth Hospital Birmingham, Birmingham, UK

Dr Manuel F. Ugarte-Gil

Hospital Guillermo Almenara Irigoyen, EsSalud, Lima, Peru

Abbreviations

ACR	American College of Rheumatology
6-MP	6-mercaptopurine
ACC	American College of Cardiology
ACIP	Advisory Committee on Immunization Practices (USA)
AHA	American Heart Association
ALMS	Aspreva Lupus Management Study
ALP	alkaline phosphatase
ALT	alanine amino transferase
ANA	antinuclear antibodies
anti-Sm	anti-Smith antibodies
apoA-1	apolipoprotein A-1
APPLE	Atherosclerosis Prevention in Pediatric Lupus Erythematosus
APRIL	a proliferation-inducing ligand
APS	antiphospholipid syndrome
APTT	activated partial thromboplastin time
AST	aspartate aminotransferase
AutoAb	autoantibody
BAFF	B cell activating factor
BAL	bronchoalveolar lavage
BCMA	B cell maturation antigen
BICLA	BILAG-based composite lupus assessment
BILAG	British Isles Lupus Assessment Group
BLyS	B lymphocyte stimulator inhibitor
BMD	bone mineral density
BMI	body mass index
Breg	B-regulatory (cell)
CAPS	catastrophic antiphospholipid syndrome
CCP	cyclic citrullinated peptide
CI	confidence interval
CIMT	carotid intima-media thickness
CIN	cervical intraepithelial neoplasia
CK	creatine kinase
CKD	chronic kidney disease
CLASI	cutaneous lupus erythematosus disease area and severity index

CMV	cytomegalovirus
CNS	central nervous system
CPRD	Clinical Practice Research Datalink
CPTA	computerized tomographic pulmonary angiography
CRP	C-reactive protein
CSF	cerebrospinal fluid
DICO	diffusion capacity for CO
DMARD	disease-modifying, anti-rheumatic drugs
DNA	deoxyribonucleic acid
dsDNA	double stranded DNA
DXA	dual-energy X-ray absorptiometry
EEG	electroencephalogram
eGFR	estimated glomerular filtration rate
ELISA	enzyme-linked immunosorbent assay
EMG	electromyography
ENA	extractable nuclear antigen
ERα	oestrogen receptor alpha
ERβ	oestrogen receptor beta
ESR	erythrocyte sedimentation rate
ESRD	end-stage renal disease
EULAR	European League Against Rheumatism
FDA	Federal Drug Administration (USA)
FEV1	forced expiratory volume in one second
FRAX	fracture risk assessment tool
FVC	forced vital capacity
GGT	gamma-glutamyl transferase
GLADEL	Grupo Latinoamericano de Estudio del Lupus
GP	general practitioner
GPRD	General Practice Research Database
GWAS	genome-wide association studies
HDL	high-density lipoprotein
HIV	human immunodeficiency virus
HLA	human leucocyte antigen
HPV	human papilloma virus
IC	immune complex
ICOS	inducible co-stimulatory molecule
IFN	interferon
IIFA	indirect immunofluorescence assay
IL	interleukin
ILD	interstitial lung disease

IRG	interferon-related genes
ISN	International Society of Nephrology
ITP	immune thrombocytopenic purpura
IVIG	intravenous immune globulin
JNC	Joint National Committee
JSLE	juvenile-onset systemic lupus erythematous
LDL	low-density lipoprotein
LE	lupus erythematosus
LMWH	low molecular weight heparin
LUMINA	LUpus in MInorities, NAture versus nurture
MAS	macrophage activation syndrome
MHC	major histocompatibility complex
MMR	measles, mumps, and rubella
MRI	magnetic resonance imaging
NET	neutrophil extracellular traps
NF-κB	nuclear factor-kappaB
NICE	National Institute for Health and Care Excellence
NP-lupus	neuro-psychiatric lupus
NSAID	non-steroidal anti-inflammatory drug
PAH	pulmonary arterial hypertension
PCR	protein:creatinine ratio
pDC	plasmacytoid dendritic cells
PET	positron emission tomography
PJP	Pneumocystis jirovecii pneumonia
PLLR	Pregnancy and Lactation Labelling Rule
PML	progressive, multifocal, leucoencephalopathy
PMN	polymorphonuclear leucocyte
PRINTO	Paediatric Rheumatology International Trials Organisation
RCT	randomized control study
RNA	ribonucleic acid
RNP	ribonucleoprotein
RPS	Renal Pathology Society
SD	standard deviation
SDI	SLICC/ACR damage index
SELENA	Safety of Estrogens in Lupus Erythematosus National Assessment
SES	social and economic status
SLAM-R	systemic lupus activity measure-revised
SLE	systemic lupus erythematosus
SLEDAI	systemic lupus erythematosus disease activity index
SLICC	Systemic Lupus International Collaborating Clinics

SMR	standardized mortality ratio
SNP	single nucleotide polymorphism
SPECT	single photon emission computerized tomography
SRI	SLE responder index
T4	thyroxine
TACI	transmembrane activator and calcium modulating ligand interactor
TAM	tyro 3, axl, mer
TB	tuberculosis
Tfh	follicular helper T cell
Th1	T-helper cell type 1
TLR	toll-like receptor
TNF	tumour necrosis factor
Treg	T-regulatory (cell)
TSH	thyroid stimulating hormone
TTP	thrombotic thrombocytopenic purpura
UK	United Kingdom
USA	United States of America
UV	ultraviolet

Chapter 1

History of systemic lupus erythematosus

Manuel F. Ugarte-Gil and Graciela S. Alarcón

> **Key points**
>
> - The first time the term lupus was used in the English literature was in the tenth century by Hebernus of Tours.
> - The first description of the systemic nature of lupus was reported by Kaposi in 1872.
> - The first description of the relapsing/remitting course of lupus was made by Osler between 1895 and 1904.
> - The description of LE cells by Hargraves (1948); the first murine model by Helyer (1963); and the studies of familial aggregation by Leonhardt (1964) and Morteo (1961) were the first steps towards understanding the pathogenesis of lupus.
> - Classification criteria for lupus were first proposed in 1971 by the American College of Rheumatology (then the American Rheumatism Association).
> - Glucocorticoids, the cornerstone in the treatment of lupus, were first used and reported by Hench in 1950. The first randomized clinical trial using cyclophosphamide was conducted at the National Institutes of Health (US) and reported in 1971.
> - Survival analyses in lupus were first reported by Merrell and Shulman in 1955; the four-year survival was 51%.
> - Non-Caucasian racial/ethnic groups experience lupus more frequently, have a more severe disease, and have worse outcomes.

Introduction

Systemic lupus erythematosus (SLE) is a chronic, relapsing, multisystemic autoimmune disorder with protean manifestations in which almost any organ system can be affected. The absence of a unique presentation makes its diagnosis difficult, even for qualified clinicians. For the purpose of this review, we have divided the history of SLE into classic, neoclassic, modern, and contemporary periods.

Classic period

Hippocrates described cutaneous ulcerations calling them *herpes esthiomenos*; it has been proposed that SLE was included under this term. However, the first time the term lupus was used in the English literature was in the tenth century by Hebernus of Tours in his *Miracles of St. Martin*; he described the healing of Eraclius, bishop of Liège who was suffering from lupus, a serious disease. The term 'lupus', however, was not systematically used for many years; and according to Virchow, Rogerius Frugardi (1230 AD) and Giovanni Manardi (1530 AD) used the term to refer to ulcers and boils in the lower extremities; facial ulcers were included in *noli me tangere* and *herpes esthiomenos*.

Two centuries later, Robert Willan (1790) presented his classification of skin diseases, *Manual of Skin Diseases*; herpes included vesicular diseases, and lupus included destructive or ulcerative skin diseases of the face and nose.

In the nineteenth century we find the first descriptions of what we now define as cutaneous lupus. Pierre Cazenave and Henry Schedel, pupils of Laurent Theodore Biett, published *Abrégé Partique Des Maladies De La Peu*, including Biett's observations. According to them, lupus should be divided into lupus which destroys only the superficial layers of the skin; lupus which destroys the deeper layers; and lupus with hypertrophy. In addition, they described *erythema centrifugum* (1833)—which is the first description of lupus erythematosus—as a rare disease which occurred more frequently among young women. The lesions occurred in the face, in the form of elevated red round patches which in cases may involve almost the entire face.

Ferdinand von Hebra, in 1846, under the heading of *seborrhea congestiva*, described two types of lesions of lupus erythematosus, one of round discs and another of confluent smaller lesions. Furthermore, he described for the first time the butterfly distribution of the facial rash—that is involving cheeks and nose. Paintings from Cazenave and von Hebra are shown in Figure 1.1.

Neoclassic period

The systemic nature of lupus was first described by Kaposi in 1872; he stated that lupus may not only extend locally, but that it also may be associated with several constitutional symptoms, such as nodules, adenitis, fever, weight loss, and arthralgias/arthritis. Furthermore, he distinguished the discoid form from lupus erythematosus *disseminatus et aggregatus*. Between 1895 and 1904, Sir William Osler described 29 patients with disparate systemic illnesses with erythema; two of them seemed to have had SLE. He, however, recognized the relapsing/remitting nature of those diseases and that systemic manifestations might occur with skin disease.

Jadassohn, in 1904, discussed both the discoid and systemic forms of lupus, including sections not only about their clinical features, but also about their pathology, aetiopathogenesis, diagnosis, prognosis, and treatment.

Emanuel Libman and Benjamin Sacks described four patients with noninfectious endocarditis, some of them with facial eruptions and kidney involvement; they considered that these patients presented similarities with the erythema group of Osler; however, they did not diagnose these patients as having SLE. Nevertheless this is now recognized as Libman–Sacks endocarditis. Baehr, Klemperer, and Schifrin (1935), in a necropsy study involving 23 SLE patients described a different type of nephritis as follows: ... *the thickened wall appears rigid, as if made of heavy wire. We have, therefore, called it the 'wire loops lesion'*. Klemperer, Pollack, and Baehr (1942) proposed that the heterogeneous organ lesions observed were due to an alteration of the collagenous tissues; based on such an assumption they recommended the term *diffuse collagen disease* for SLE and systemic sclerosis.

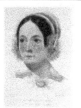

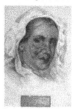

Fig.1: "Seborrhoea congestiva", Dr. Anton Elfinger, Vienna 1845

From Biett (1781-1840) to Dohi (1866-1931):Iconography of Lupus erythematosus (LE).

Stella Fatovic-Ferencic*, Karl Holubar**, Depts. of History of Medicine, Croatian Acad Sci & Arts, Zagreb Croatia*, Univ of Vienna, Vienna Austria**

Lupus *erythematosus* by today has replaced Lupus *vulgaris* as the more frequent disorder labeld with this term. Historically, *lupus* means a destructive process leading to tissue defects in consequence. The 19th century with its rise of tuberculosis in the industrial urban centers brought skin tuberculosis (lupus vulgaris is one form of it) in front. First described by Biett as *Erythème centrifuge*, LE appeared in medical literature already around mid 1850[1,2].The picture given in the book on Biett's teachings is L. vulgaris however[2].

The 19th century was the heyday of dermatological illustration by hand, i.e. painting, lithographies and moulages. Beginning with JL Alibert's atlas (1806-1814) and MN Devergie's, 'a series of grand-format publications started to appear which lasted into the early years of this century, WJE Wilson[3], PLA Cazenave[4], F Hebra[5], , R Taylor[6], R Crocker[7], P. Morrow[8], to name but a few. Eventually Keizo Dohi's[9], was the first atlas from outside the Euro-American sphere (1903-1910). At the end of this development moulages, as individual, three dimensional colored replicas of a patients' pathology and photographs replaced paintings. The picture series illustrates the change of style, from elegant portraits to frugal pictorial demonstration of disease. (Figures relate to refs. #3-9 and the oeuvre of Hebra's two painter physicians).

(1) Cazenave (A): Revue clinique hebdomadaire. La Lancette Française: Gazette des Hôpitaux civils et militaires Samedi 27 Juillet 1850. p.354 col 3, para 3, lines 15-20

(2) Cazenave A and Schedel HE: Abrégé pratique des maladies de la peau. Paris, Bechet Jeune 1828 and 1838 (1st and 2nd ed.)

(3) Wilson WJE: Portraits of diseases of the skin, London 1855

(4) Cazenave PKA: Leçons sur les maladies de la peau, Paris 1856

(5) Hebra F: Atlas der Hautkrankheiten, Wien 1856-76

(6) Taylor RW: A clinical atlas of venereal and skin diseases Philadelphia 1889

(7) Crocker HR: Atlas of the diseases of the skin, London 1903

(8) Besnier E Fournier A et al: Le Musée de l'Hôpital Saint-Louis, Paris 1894?

(9) Dohi K: Atlas der Hautkrankheiten. Tokyo 1903-10

Acknowledgments:A. Weissenbach MA, K. Stockl

Fig.2: "Inflammatio Adfectuum", William Bagg, London ref.#6

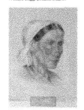

Fig.3: Lupus erythematosus, Dr. Anton Elfinger, Vienna, ref.#5

Fig.5: Lupus erythematosus, Vittoria-Gabriel or Marie-Firmin Bocourt, Paris, ref.#4

Fig.6: Lupus erythematosus generalisatus, Dr. Carl Heitzmann Vienna

Fig.7: Lupus erythematosus, Tregord Bill ?, London, ref.#7

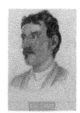

Fig.8: Lupus erythematosus, Dr. Julius Heitzmann, Vienna

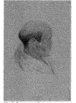

Fig.9: Lupus erythematosus, photographed from a facsimile edition unknown painter, Tokyo, ref.#9

GAZETTE DES HOPITAUX
CIVILS ET MILITAIRES

Fig.11: First mentioned of the term Lupus érythémateux in July 1850 by PLA Cazenave, Paris ref. #1

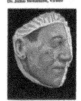

Fig.10: Lupus erythematosus, Moulage by John Baretta, Paris, ref.#8

Figure 1.1 From Biett (1781–1840) to Dohi (1866–1931). Iconography of lupus erythematosus.

3

Modern period

The discovery of lupus erythematosus (LE) cell by Hargraves et al. in 1948 undoubtedly was the departing point toward our understanding of SLE. They described cells which they named LE cells in bone marrow preparations from patients with SLE; according to them these cells represented:

> . . . the end result of one of two things: either phagocytosis of free nuclear material with a resulting round vacuole containing this partially digested and lysed nuclear material, or, second, an actual autolysis of one or more of lobes of the nucleus of the involved cell so that it presents essentially the same appearance as the one which has phagocytized nuclear material . . .

An LE cell is shown in Figure 1.2. Haserick in 1950 showed that the serum factor responsible for the LE cell was a gamma globulin. Over the next ten years, Friou (1958) and Holman et al. (1959) described that globulins from the sera of SLE patients were directed to DNA or histones. Moore and Lutz (1955) found that patients with false-positive serological tests for syphilis were at an increased risk for having or developing SLE or diseases similar to SLE.

Another important milestone was the discovery of kidney disease in the New Zealand black/white F1 hybrid mouse (NZB/NZW F1). This mouse developed a disease similar to SLE with haematological involvement, antinuclear antibodies, and glomerulonephritis. This and other murine models have allowed us to understand immune tolerance, the development of autoantibodies, the pathogenesis of some clinical manifestations, such as glomerulonephritis, and the recognition of possible targets for drug development.

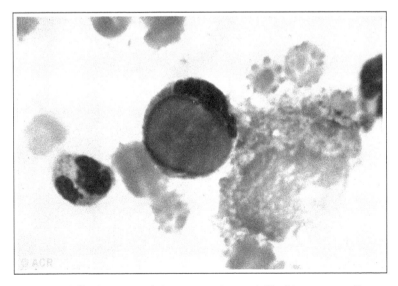

Figure 1.2 LE cell: This photomicrograph demonstrates a characteristic LE cell that was prepared from peripheral blood of a patient with systemic lupus erythematosus. A homogeneous inclusion is present in a polymorphonuclear leukocyte.

Understanding of the importance of genetic factors in SLE began to develop over the next few years, aided by familial aggregation studies such as the ones conducted in Mälmo (Leonhardt, 1964) and New York (Morteo, 1961); taken together, these studies suggested the importance of familial aggregation in SLE, but also the influence of environmental factors in the course of SLE. Subsequently, Arnett and Shulman described an average difference in the age at onset of SLE of nine years in siblings and of two years in identical twins, suggesting that environmental factors influence the initiation of SLE.

To produce a definition of SLE that allowed patients to be classified for epidemiological, clinical, or therapeutic studies, criteria were established by a Committee of the American Rheumatism Association, now the American College of Rheumatology (ACR). The first set of criteria were proposed in 1971, whereby a patient was considered to have SLE if four of 14 criteria were present; these criteria were revised and reduced to 11 in 1982, but still four were needed. Fifteen years later, these criteria were updated (but never validated), replacing the positive LE cells for the antiphospholipid antibodies.

As the understanding of SLE increased it was felt necessary to measure disease changes. Several disease activity indices have been proposed over the years but the ones most frequently used nowadays are the systemic lupus erythematosus disease activity index (SLEDAI) and its variants, and the British Isles Lupus Assessment Group (BILAG) and its variants. Another important outcome of SLE is the occurrence of organ damage due to disease activity, treatment, and/or comorbidities; damage is evaluated with the Systemic Lupus International Collaborating Clinics (SLICC)/ACR damage index (SDI) developed in 1996, which includes irreversible changes occurring in 12 organ/systems after SLE diagnosis.

Cortisone, the cornerstone in the management of several autoimmune diseases was first used in SLE in 1950 by Hench, resulting in the improvement of clinical manifestations. Steinberg, in 1971, conducted a clinical trial on 13 patients with lupus nephritis, finding that cyclophosphamide improved urinary sediment, proteinuria, immunological activity, and extrarenal disease. Several studies followed corroborating the efficacy of cyclophosphamide in SLE. Antimalarials are now recommended for every SLE patient, unless a major contraindication exists, since it has proven to have several beneficial effects in these patients, including a decrease in the probability of flare-ups, in the occurrence of damage, and on early mortality. However, it is worth pointing out that quinine had been reported to be useful in SLE as early as 1894 by Payne, as reported by Leden.

Survival analyses in SLE were first reported by Merrell and Shulman in 1955 who found a 51% 4-year survival probability. Survival in SLE has improved steadily since then; by the end of the twentieth century, the 20-year survival was 68%. However, it has been recognized that, by and large, non-Caucasian ethnic/racial groups not only experience SLE more frequently—as shown by Fessel, who in 1974 reported lupus as occurring more frequently among black women—but as a more severe disease, with worse outcomes and greater damage accrual. For example, compared with Caucasians, Hispanics, Asians, and African descendants accrue more damage. Survival is also lower among non-Caucasians; however, when socioeconomic factors were included in the analyses, ethnicity did not remain associated with survival, with the exception of the study from the Duke's cohort.

Contemporary period: SLE in the twenty-first century

In the twenty-first century our understanding of the pathogenesis of SLE is rapidly unravelling as fruitful collaborations among investigators across the world are established and current technologies allow studies to be conducted. Genetic studies have allowed the recognition of a number of markers associated with several pathways involved in SLE pathogenesis such as DNA degradation, apoptosis, type I interferon, toll-like receptors, and nuclear factor-kappaB (NF-κB) signalling, immune-complex processing and phagocytosis, as well as B and T cells, neutrophils, and monocyte function and signalling. In parallel, several environmental factors which may trigger or worsen SLE have been recognized, including ultraviolet light, vitamin D deficiency, smoking, and chemicals such as silica or mercury.

Recently, the SLICC group has published a new set of criteria which include manifestations not present in the previous ones; with these criteria, a patient must satisfy at least four including at least one clinical and one immunologic criterion, or a biopsy-proven lupus nephritis with antinuclear antibodies or anti-double stranded DNA antibodies.

As our understanding of the pathogenesis of SLE improves, targeted new treatments have been and are being developed; the first biologic therapy for SLE, belimumab, was the first drug approved by the FDA for SLE patients in more than 50 years.

Further reading

Abu-Shakra M, Urowitz MB, Gladman DD, Gough J. Mortality studies in systemic lupus erythematosus. Results from a single center. II. Predictor variables for mortality. *J Rheumatol* 1995;22:1265–70.

Arnett FC, Shulman LE. Studies in familial systemic lupus erythematosus. *Medicine* (Baltimore) 1976;55:313–22.

Baehr G, Klemperer P, Schifrin A. A diffuse disease of the peripheral circulation (usually associated with lupus erythematosus and endocarditis). *Am J Med* 1952;13:591–6.

Cohen A, Reynolds W, Franklin E, et al. Diagnostic and therapeutic criteria committee of The American Rheumatism Association. Preliminary criteria for the classification of systemic lupuserythematosus. *Bull Rheum Dis* 1971;21:643.

Fessel WJ. Systemic lupus erythematosus in the community. Incidence, prevalence, outcome, and first symptoms; the high prevalence in black women. *Arch Intern Med* 1974;134:1027–35.

Hargraves MM, Richmond H, Morton R. Presentation of two bone marrow elements; the tart cell and the LE cell. *Proc Staff Meet Mayo Clin* 1948;23:25–8.

Helyer BJ, Howie JB. Spontaneous auto-immune disease in NZB/BL mice. *Br J Haematol* 1963;9:119–31.

Hench PS, Kendall EC, Slocumb CH, Polley HF. Effects of cortisone acetate and pituitary ACTH on rheumatoid arthritis, rheumatic fever and certain other conditions. *Arch Intern Med* 1950;85:545–666.

Holubar K. Terminology and iconography of lupus erythematosus. A historical vignette. *Am J Dermatopathol* 1980;2:239–42.

Klemperer P, Pollack AD, Baehr G. Landmark article May 23, 1942: Diffuse collagen disease. Acute disseminated lupus erythematosus and diffuse scleroderma. *JAMA* 1984;251:1593–4.

Leden I. Antimalarial drugs-350 years. *Scand J Rheumatol* 1981;10:307–12.

Libman E, Sacks B. A hitherto undescribed form of valvular and mural endocarditis. *Trans Assoc Am Phys* 1923;38:46–61.

Merrell M, Shulman LE. Determination of prognosis in chronic disease, illustrated by systemic lupus erythematosus. *J Chronic Dis* 1955;1:12–32.

Smith CD, Cyr M. The history of lupus erythematosus. From Hippocrates to Osler. *Rheum Dis Clin North Am* 1988;14:1–14.

Steinberg AD, Kaltreider HB, Staples PJ, Goetzl EJ, Talal N, Decker JL. Cyclophosphamide in lupus nephritis: a controlled trial. *Ann Intern Med* 1971;75:165–71.

Chapter 2

Aetiopathogenesis of systemic lupus erythematosus

Peter Lloyd, Sarah Doaty, and Bevra H. Hahn

Key points

- The pathogenesis of lupus is characterized by a complex interplay of genetic predisposition and environmental exposures, loss of immune tolerance, and immune activation.
- Autoantibodies play a role in tissue damage in SLE patients; some are useful markers for diagnosis and monitoring of disease.
- Defects in innate immunity that contribute to the pathogenesis of SLE include deficiencies of and/or increased activation of complement; abnormal phagocytosis and activation of monocytes; up-regulation of toll-like receptors (TLRs) on dendritic cells and B cells; and abnormal NETosis in low-density granulocytes.
- Loss of self-tolerance within the adaptive immune system leads to the production of autoantibodies, without the usual regulation, in patients with pre-clinical and active SLE.
- There are very few single 'lupus genes' and they are rare. Most affected individuals with SLE inherit multiple gene polymorphisms that are normal.
- UV light, silica dust, and certain infections have all been implicated in the pathogenesis of SLE.
- Women of childbearing age are nine times more likely than men to develop SLE, and contributing factors may include higher levels of oestradiol, abnormal methylation of genes/gene regions on the suppressed X chromosome, and exposure to silica dust.

Introduction

Systemic lupus erythematosus (SLE) is an autoimmune disease characterized by the presence of autoreactive B and T cells and the production of a broad, heterogeneous group of autoantibodies (autoAb).[1] The pathogenesis of lupus can be divided into three stages: 1) genetic predisposition and environmental exposures, 2) loss of tolerance, and 3) immune activation. In stage one, there is a long period of predisposition to autoimmunity with genetic susceptibility and environmental exposures each contributing to disease development. More than fifty genes have been associated with SLE. Sex also plays a role in disease susceptibility, as women of child-bearing age are nine times more likely than men to develop SLE.[2] Environmental factors, such as ultraviolet light exposure, and exposure to infection, such as that of Epstein–Barr virus, have been suspected

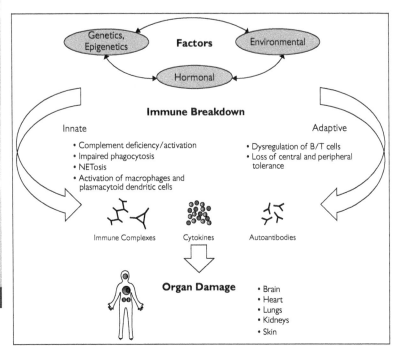

Figure 2.1 Overview of pathogenesis of SLE.

as inducers or enhancers of SLE.[2] Stage two develops when there is a loss of tolerance to self-antigens, and autoAb are generated. The third and final stage is inadequate regulation of autoAb production with T and B cells hyperactivated, and innate immune systems also programmed toward inflammation eventually leading to tissue damage and clinical manifestations of disease.[2] The pathogenesis of SLE is summarized in Figure 2.1.

Autoantibodies

In patients with SLE, autoantibodies are the main effectors of disease onset.[2] Pathogenic subsets of autoAb and immune complexes (IC), deposited in or on tissues activate complement, with release of cytokines, chemokines, and proteolytic enzymes, resulting in organ inflammation, cell death, and tissue damage.[2] Autoantibodies precede the first symptoms of disease by an average of 2–3 years in 85% of SLE patients with some reports showing up to 9 years.[2] The specificity and expression of autoAb can vary over time, for example anti-dsDNA and anti-C1q levels correlate with activity of lupus nephritis, whereas anti-Smith (anti-Sm) levels usually remain stable in an individual through the course of their disease.[3] Over 140 autoAb have been identified and associated with rheumatic diseases. We will discuss those autoAb relevant to the pathogenesis of SLE. In SLE patients there is a temporal hierarchy of expression of autoAb with antinuclear antibodies (ANA) appearing first, followed by anti-DNA and antiphospholipid antibodies, which are then followed by anti-Smith (anti-Sm) and anti-ribonucleoprotein antibodies (anti-RNP).[2] (See Table 2.1 Autoantibodies in lupus)

Table 2.1 Autoantibodies in systemic lupus erythematosus				
Autoantibodies	Specificity/sensitivity in SLE (%)	Prevalence in SLE (%)	Clinical relevance	Other disease associations
ANA	High specificity Low sensitivity	>95	ACR and SLICC criteria.	Mixed connective tissue disease, scleroderma, Sjogren's syndrome, rheumatoid arthritis, polymyositis, dermatomyositis, drug-induced LE, infections, malignancy, medications
dsDNA	High specificity Medium sensitivity	70–98	ACR and SLICC criteria.	Rare in other rheumatic diseases
Anti-nucleosome	High specificity High sensitivity	85	Lupus nephritis	Autoimmune hepatitis, mixed connective tissue disease, scleroderma, Sjogren's syndrome
Anti-SSA/Ro	Moderate specificity Moderate sensitivity	25	Sicca symptoms, subacute cutaneous SLE, pneumonitis, shrinking lung syndrome, thrombocytopenia, lymphopenia, nephritis, vasculitis, thrombocytopenic purpura, ocular damage, congenital heart block, skin rash in newborn	Sjogren's syndrome, rheumatoid arthritis, polymyositis, scleroderma
Anti-SSB/La	Moderate specificity Moderate sensitivity	10–15	Congenital heart block	Sjogren's syndrome
Anti-Smith	High specificity Low sensitivity	30	ACR criteria; mortality, serositis, nephritis, neuropsychiatric SLE, pulmonary fibrosis, leucopenia, arthritis, malar rash, discoid rash, vasculitis, pulmonary hypertension, peripheral neuropathy	Rare in other autoimmune diseases

(continued)

Table 2.1 Continued

Autoantibodies	Specificity/sensitivity in SLE (%)	Prevalence in SLE (%)	Clinical relevance	Other disease associations
Anti-U1-RNP		25	Interstitial lung disease, rapid progression pulmonary damage, pleuritis, neuropsychiatric LE, Raynaud's phenomenon, leucopenia, meningitis, arthritis, fevers, myositis	Mixed connective tissue disease, scleroderma, polymyositis, rheumatoid arthritis, Sjogren's syndrome
Anti-ribosomal P	Moderate specificity Moderate sensitivity	10–40	Neuropsychiatric LE, hepatitis	
Anti-phospholipids	Low specificity Low sensitivity	30–40	Thrombocytopenia, clotting, fetal loss	Malignancy, infection, medication-induced
Anti-C1q	Low specificity Low sensitivity	33	Nephritis	hypocomplementaemic urticarial vasculitis, rheumatoid arthritis, Felty's syndrome, rheumatoid vasculitis, Sjogren's syndrome
Anti-histone	Low specificity Low sensitivity	70–80	Drug-induced LE	Scleroderma, rheumatoid arthritis, Felty's syndrome, Sjogren's syndrome, juvenile rheumatoid arthritis, mixed connective tissue disease, vasculitis, malignancy, liver disease

Abbreviations: ACR: American College of Rheumatology; LE: lupus erythematosus; SLICC: Systemic Lupus International Collaborating Clinics.

Antinuclear antibodies

Antinuclear antibodies are directed at various cellular compartments including: nuclear constituents, components of the nuclear envelope, mitotic spindle apparatus, cytosol, cytoplasmic organelles and cell membranes.[2] Antinuclear antibodies can be detected by several types of assays, the most commonly used include the indirect immunofluorescence assay (IIFA) and the enzyme-linked immunosorbent assay (ELISA). The indirect immunofluorescence assay uses cultured cells as substrates and is considered the criterion standard by the American College of Rheumatology; it is recommended as the most accurate, reproducible assay. The fluorescence pattern appearance may be homogeneous, speckled, nucleolar, centromere, atypical, or peripheral. A homogeneous pattern suggests SLE; speckled is nonspecific; and nucleolar or centromere patterns suggest scleroderma. The ANA titre is the highest serum dilution factor at which fluorescence can be observed. The higher the titre of ANA, the higher the probability for the presence of rheumatic disease. Antinuclear antibodies are present in about 95% of SLE patients with active disease.[1] Not all antinuclear antibodies are pathogenic. A recent study showed that 13.8% of the normal population was ANA positive, with the frequency higher in women than men.[2] What is challenging for the physician today, is attempting to distinguish among these individuals who are destined to develop disease and those who will not. One must also remember that there are other non-rheumatic causes of a positive ANA such as infections (tuberculosis, malaria, syphilis, acute and chronic viral syndromes, etc.), malignancies (hepatocellular carcinoma, malignant melanoma, and leukaemia/lymphoma) and several medications (hydralazine, procainamide, isoniazid, chlorpromazine, interferons, TNF inhibitors, minocycline, anticonvulsants, lithium, and methyldopa).

Anti-DNA antibodies

Anti-DNA antibodies constitute a subgroup of antinuclear antibodies that bind to either single-stranded or double-stranded DNA (dsDNA). Double-stranded DNA antibodies can be found in up to 70–80% of patients with SLE during the course of their disease.[2] Anti-dsDNA antibodies are included in the American College of Rheumatology classification criteria and the Systemic Lupus International Collaborating Clinics (SLICC) criteria for SLE. In a majority of patients, there is a relationship between disease activity and the serum titre of anti-dsDNA.[2] Several studies have looked at pre-emptive treatment with corticosteroids for patients with rising dsDNA and falling complement levels without clinical signs of SLE activity. Treatment reduced flare rates, but some patients exposed to treatment would not have flared.[2] There is a small group of SLE patients who have a persistently elevated anti-dsDNA without any significant disease activity, known as serologically active, but clinically quiescent SLE.[2] The anti-dsDNA antibody titre is measured by an ELISA or Crithidia luciliae immunofluorescence assay.[2] There are several theories on how anti-dsDNA antibodies bind to tissue, activate complement, and cause inflammation. Initial theories proposed that anti-dsDNA forms complexes with free floating dsDNA or nucleosomes and is then deposited in various tissues.[2] More recent data suggest that complexes are formed between nucleosome fragments and anti-dsDNA antibodies as there is little free floating dsDNA in human serum.[2] In any individual, oligonucleosome debris is formed as a normal by-product of cellular breakdown. In SLE patients the removal of this apoptotic debris is known to be slower, allowing for more circulating nucleosome material to induce and interact with anti-dsDNA antibodies.[2]

Anti-nucleosome antibodies

A nucleosome consists of DNA wrapped around a histone octomer.[2] Anti-nucleosome antibodies were the first ANAs described in SLE. Anti-nucleosomes are present in approximately 85% of SLE patients.[1] Anti-nucleosome antibodies are also found in 40–50% of patients with autoimmune hepatitis, and to a lesser extent in patients with mixed connective tissue disease, systemic sclerosis, and Sjogren's syndrome.[2] They correlate roughly with lupus nephritis, but probably not as well as anti-dsDNA and anti-C1q.

Anti-SSA/Ro antibodies

The SSA/Ro antigens are ribonucleoproteins containing small uridine-rich nucleic acids.[1] The approximate prevalence of Anti-SSA/Ro in SLE patients is 25% (25–60%).[2] Anti-SSA/Ro antibodies can also be seen in Sjogren's syndrome (60–90%), rheumatoid arthritis, polymyositis, and systemic sclerosis.[2] Patients with anti-SSA/Ro antibodies are at increased risk for: sicca symptoms, photosensitive skin rash (subacute cutaneous lupus), pneumonitis, shrinking lung syndrome, thrombocytopenia, lymphopenia, nephritis, vasculitis, thrombocytopenic purpura, ocular damage, secondary Sjogren's syndrome, and QT prolongation.[2] Anti-SSA/Ro antibodies can cross the placenta resulting in neonatal lupus. Both anti-SSA/Ro and anti-SSB/La antibodies can bind to the fetal heart conduction system, inhibit cardiac repolarization, and cause complete atrioventricular block.[1] Complete atrioventricular heart block occurs in approximately 1–2% of pregnancies; this increases to 15% of any subsequent pregnancies in mothers who have already given birth to a child with congenital heart block.[4] Neonatal lupus dermatitis usually subsides once the maternal antibodies are cleared from the infants circulation at 6–12 months (2), but cardiac involvement sometimes progresses to severe myocardiopathy.[2]

Anti-SSB/La antibodies

The SSB/La antigen is a phosphoprotein that binds a variety of small RNAs, including 5S cellular RNA, transfer RNA, 7S RNA, and hY RNA.[2] The approximate prevalence of Anti-SSB/La in patients with SLE is 10–15%, and 30–60% in patients with primary Sjogren's syndrome.[2] Anti-SSB/La antibodies are almost always found with anti-SSA/Ro antibodies, whereas SSA/Ro antibodies are often present without SSB/La antibodies.[2]

Anti-Smith antibodies (anti-Sm)

Anti-Sm antibodies react to several antigens in small ribonucleoprotein particles.[2] Anti-Sm antibodies are a highly specific marker for SLE.[1] The approximate prevalence of anti-Sm is about 30% among black patients, but varies significantly across different ethnic groups, with only 10% prevalence in Caucasians.[2] Anti-Sm positivity is included in the American College of Rheumatology classification criteria and SLICC criteria for SLE. Anti-Sm expression is generally persistent throughout the disease course and there does not seem to be a correlation between titres and disease activity.[1] Patients with anti-Sm antibodies are at increased risk for: mortality, serositis, lupus nephritis, neuropsychiatric lupus, pulmonary fibrosis, leucopenia, arthritis, malar and discoid rash, vasculitis, peripheral neuropathy, and pulmonary hypertension.[2]

Anti-U1-RNP antibodies

Anti-RNP antibodies are directed towards small nuclear ribonucleoprotein particles that are different from anti-Sm specificities.[2] The approximate prevalence of Anti-U1-RNP antibodies in SLE patients is 25% (13–47%).[2] Like anti-Sm antibodies, there is significant variation in prevalence across different ethnic groups. Anti-U1-RNP antibodies are more common in African American SLE patients.[2] Anti-U1-RNP antibodies are not used to confirm a diagnosis of SLE due to the low sensitivity and specificity. These antibodies are also seen in mixed connective tissue disease, scleroderma, polymyositis, rheumatoid arthritis, and Sjogren's syndrome.[1] Patients with anti-U1-RNP antibodies are at increased risk for: interstitial lung disease, rapid progression of pulmonary damage, pleuritis, central nervous system (CNS) involvement, Raynaud's phenomenon, leucopenia, meningitis, older age at disease onset, arthritis, erosive joint disease, fevers, and myositis.[2]

Anti-ribosomal P antibodies

The anti-ribosomal antigens are three highly conserved phosphorylated proteins located on the 60S-ribosomal subunit in the cell cytoplasm.[1] The prevalence of serum anti-P antibody varies from 10% with inactive disease to 40% in active disease.[2] Despite the low prevalence there is very high specificity of up to 90% for SLE.[2] Some, but not all, studies suggest that anti-ribosomal P antibodies are associated with malar rash, oral ulcer, photosensitivity, lupus nephritis, neuropsychiatric lupus (including depression), and SLE-associated hepatitis.[5]

Anti-phospholipid antibodies

Anti-phospholipid antibodies are seen in 30–40% of SLE patients.[1] Anti-phospholipid antibodies include: lupus anticoagulant, anti-cardiolipin antibodies, and anti-β2-glycoprotein antibodies. Only one third of patients with SLE and anti-phospholipid antibodies will at some point during their disease develop clinical symptoms due to the anti-phospholipid antibodies.[2] Anti-phospholipid antibodies are also seen in other autoimmune diseases, infections, malignancies, drug-induced disorders, and healthy individuals.[1] Antiphospholipid syndrome (APS) is an acquired thrombophilia characterized by vascular thrombosis (venous, arterial, or small vessel) and/or fetal morbidity in utero.[2] Antiphospholipid syndrome can be a primary disorder or a secondary disorder such as in SLE.[2] To meet classification criteria for either primary or secondary APS, antibodies must be present on two separate occasions separated by at least 12 weeks, and the patient must have a thrombotic episode and/or multiple fetal losses.[2]

Anti-C1q antibodies

C1q is a cationic glycoprotein of 410–450 kDa, which binds to the Fc portions of immunoglobulins in immune complexes leading to complement activation.[1] Anti C1q antibodies are found in 17–46% of SLE patients.[1] C1q acts as a binding molecule between debris from cellular apoptosis and macrophages.[1] This suggests that the development of anti-C1q antibodies may be related to the slower rate of apoptotic cellular debris removal in SLE patients.[1] Anti-C1q antibodies are not limited to SLE and are present in almost 100% of patients with hypocomplementaemic urticarial vasculitis.[2] Other conditions that can have positive anti-C1q antibodies include: rheumatoid arthritis, Felty's syndrome, rheumatoid vasculitis, and Sjogren's syndrome.[1] Anti-C1q antibodies are more prevalent in SLE patients who have proliferative lupus nephritis, 63%.[2] Some experts consider anti-C1q as good as, or better than, anti-dsDNA in predicting that a patient will develop lupus nephritis, or is about to experience a disease flare. However, the assay is not widely available in service laboratories.

Anti-histone antibodies

Anti-histone antibodies are a group of antibodies that are reactive to any of five major classes of histones (H1, H2A, H2B, H3, and H4), which organize and constrain the topology of DNA.[1] Anti-histone positivity is seen mainly in patients with drug-induced lupus, but can also be present in SLE as well as rheumatoid arthritis, malignancy, and liver disease. Drug-induced lupus erythematosus (LE) tends to be a milder disease with a lower frequency of nephritis.[2] Drug-induced LE usually remits after discontinuation of the culprit medication. Medications clearly associated with drug-induced LE include TNF inhibitors, interferons, minocycline, lithium, anticonvulsants, isoniazid, procainamide, penicillamine, and methyldopa.[1] There is limited utility in supporting a clinical diagnosis of SLE with anti-histone antibodies, and they are not in classification criteria.[2]

Anti-lipoprotein antibodies

Patients with lupus are at an increased risk of cardiovascular disease, this may be due in part to higher levels of antibodies to high-density lipoprotein (HDL) and apolipoprotein A-1 (apoA-1); both lipoproteins, when active, protect from atherosclerosis by preventing oxidation of low-density lipoprotein (LDL) and by reverse cholesterol transport.[2] Measurements of these antibodies are not widely available.

Innate immunity in SLE

The innate immune system plays a central role both in the initiation and continuation of autoimmunity in SLE patients. Normally, when IC form in circulation, or in tissues, the complement system functions to solubilize and clear the IC through the classic, alternative, and lectin pathways. Deficiency in complement components, especially C1q, has been associated with early onset of disease. Increased complement activation and consumption plays a major role in propagating disease.[6] In patients with SLE, the ability to clear IC may also be diminished due to polymorphism in Fc receptors[2], and possibly to inherent defects in phagocytic cells, particularly monocytes. Complement activation also serves to recruit inflammatory cells to the site of IC deposition with resultant inflammatory cytokine/chemokine release and tissue damage.

It is well known that there is impaired clearance of apoptotic cell debris by macrophages from some SLE patients.[2] This impaired clearance allows for apoptotic cells and debris to serve as immunogens that drive the production of autoAb.[7] Apoptotic cells are recognized by macrophages through several surface receptors.[7] A receptor that appears to be relevant to the SLE population is the tyro 3, axl, mer (TAM) receptor, which plays an important role in the clearance of apoptotic cells.[7] Murine models lacking TAM have impaired clearance of apoptotic cells and develop lupus-like autoimmunity.[7]

Toll-like receptors (TLR) constitute a family of receptors that function as sensors for microbial invaders. Toll-like receptors are located on the cell surface or within endosomes of several cell types.[7] Activation of TLR leads to the recruitment of adapter proteins, activation of protein kinases, transcription factors, expression of inflammatory cytokines (tumour necrosis factor (TNF), interleukin-1 (IL-1), and IL-12), chemokines (monocyte chemoattractant protein-1, IL-8) endothelial adhesion molecules, co-stimulatory molecules (CD80 and CD86), and antiviral cytokines (interferon alfa (IFN-α)).[7] Toll-like receptor-dependent induction of IFN-α (mostly from plasmacytoid dendritic cells, pDC) leads to further up-regulation of TLR in autoreactive B cells thus fuelling the autoimmune response.[8] Hydroxychloroquine, a modestly effective treatment for SLE, may interfere with the innate immune system by blocking the activation of two TLRs (TLR7 and TLR9), which are known to be stimulated by RNA and DNA, respectively, followed by activation of IFNα-signalling.[8]

NETosis is a form of cell death in neutrophils by which they exude a meshwork of chromatin fibres called neutrophil extracellular traps (NET) into the extracellular space, capturing foreign pathogens and cellular debris, and neutralizing pathogens via production of reactive oxygen species. Low density granulocytes, which are increased in the circulation of many patients with SLE, are particularly prone to NETosis. Residual circulating NETs promote SLE in several ways: 1) they are a source of autoantigens (capable of inducing immune responses to DNA and nucleosomes); 2) NETosing polymorphonuclear leucocytes (PMN) cause endothelial damage; 3) they increase activation of inflammasomes; 4) they activate plasmacytoid dendritic cells; and (6) plasmacytoid dendritic cells release large amounts of IFN-α, a hallmark of the inflammatory cascade in SLE (approximately 50% of SLE patients with mild disease, and 75% of patients with lupus nephritis have elevated signatures for genes induced by IFN). Through a self-perpetuating feedback loop, IFN-α increases NET production in circulating neutrophils.[9]

A well-functioning phagocytic pathway is an important factor in the prevention of autoimmunity. In patients with SLE, the phagocytic pathway is disrupted by dysfunctional monocyte-derived macrophages, leading to increased levels of circulating cellular debris and self-antigens. Phagocytic defects in patients with SLE include decreased activity, smaller size, impaired adherence, and increased apoptosis of monocyte-derived macrophages.[10] Murine models also show that tissue-fixed activated macrophages play a major role in the acute and chronic renal inflammation and fibrosis that constitutes lupus nephritis.[11]

Adaptive immunity in SLE

Fundamental to the normal immune response is recognition of self from non-self and the development of tolerance. Tolerance is the selective lack of immune response to self-targeted antigens. Both B and T cells undergo various mechanisms throughout development to achieve tolerance. Central tolerance occurs during the maturation of lymphocytes in the central (generative) lymphoid organs. Peripheral tolerance occurs as a consequence of recognizing self-antigens by mature circulating lymphocytes. In SLE there is a breakdown of tolerance at many of the various tolerance checkpoints. These breakdowns allow for the production of autoAb leading to inflammation, tissue damage, and disease. The loss of self-tolerance in SLE may be a result of genetics, epigenetics, and environmental exposures. Loss of tolerance in both T cells and B cells plays a significant role in the pathogenesis of SLE.

T cells are critical in the pathogenesis of SLE; they enhance the production of autoAb by providing help to B cells to differentiate, proliferate, and mature.[12] T cells also support the class switching of the autoAb that B cells are expressing to IgG, which is generally more pathogenic than IgM.[12] There are many mechanisms of breakdown in both central and peripheral T cell tolerance in SLE patients. Significant T cells in SLE include: T-helper cell type 1 (Th1), T-helper cell type 2 (Th2), Th17 cells, follicular T cells (Tfh) and T-regulatory (Treg) cells. T cells from SLE patients are more resistant to induction of apoptosis by thymic stromal cells.[2] Activated T cells of SLE patients resist anergy and apoptosis by up-regulating the COX-2/FLIP anti-apoptosis mechanism.[2] There is a reduction in stability and therefore an increase in degradation of CD3 subunits of T cells in SLE patients.[12] This leads to an increase in expression of FcR receptors and activation of the associated Syk pathway.[12] This alters expression of certain genes, resulting in expression of T cell CD40L—a co-stimulatory molecule which promotes B cell differentiation, proliferation, antibody production, and class switching.[12] Prior studies suggested anti-CD40L might be effective in SLE, but there were significant thromboembolic side effects in clinical trials.[13]

Defects in production of IL-2 are characteristic of T cells from SLE patients; and this alters activation pathways to skew T cell differentiation of naïve cells toward pro-inflammatory Th1, Th17, and Tfh descendants, rather than to the less inflammatory Th2 and the protective Tregs.[7,14] Th17 cells secrete IL-17.[12] IL-17 works in synergy with other cytokines such as TNFα, IL-1β, IL-22, and IFN-γ to stabilize the mRNA of pro-inflammatory cytokines and chemokines, thus promoting inflammation.[15] Follicular helper T cells, found predominantly in tissues rather than in the circulation, produce high levels of IL-21 and inducible co-stimulatory molecule (ICOS), which promote B-cell proliferation, affinity maturation, and terminal differentiation into plasma cells in lymphoid tissues, promoting autoAb formation and autoimmunity.[2,13] Lupus patients can have an elevated number of circulating Tfh cells; these numbers positively correlate with levels of autoAb, numbers of circulating B cells, and disease severity.[13] SLE T cells also have abnormalities in their lipid raft composition and dynamics.[2] Lipid rafts are critical for T cell regulation of activation pathways.[2] As helper T cells of various types are increased in function in patients with SLE, regulatory T cells are deficient either in numbers or function, or both.

There are three major distinct tolerance checkpoints in B cell development: 1) maturation of B cells in the bone marrow, 2) development in the peripheral lymphoid organs, and 3) checkpoints involving mature B cell subsets.[2] There is a 'leak' of tolerance mechanisms at several checkpoints, which can vary among SLE patients, but allows autoreactive B cells to reach the circulation and target tissues.[2] At the immature stage, a majority of autoreactive B cells either undergo clonal deletion, anergy, or receptor editing. In patients with SLE, multiple defective checkpoints have been identified at this stage.[2] Increased expression of co-stimulatory molecules seen in SLE patients can protect transitional B-cells from apoptosis.[2] In some SLE patients, elevated levels of B cell activating factor (BAFF) also known as B-lymphocyte stimulator (BLyS), a cytokine required for maturation and survival of B cells at several developmental stages, associate with rescue of self-reactive B cells from anergy and deletion.[2] Belimumab, a fully humanized monoclonal antibody that binds soluble BAFF and reduces B cell numbers, particularly in naïve groups, has been approved by the FDA for treatment of active SLE.

There can also be a defect at the germinal centre entry checkpoint in SLE. Autoreactive B cells are able to escape normal censoring allowing for the development of IgG memory and plasma cells.[2] Self-reactive B cells that avoid tolerance checkpoints throughout their transitional stages may mature to be plasmacytoid autoAb-secreting B cells of any B cell subset including: B-1 cells, marginal zone B cells, and follicular B cells.[2] Current literature suggests that marginal zone B cells and B-1a cells contribute to the production of pathogenic autoAb while B-regulatory cells (Breg or B10) suppress these responses.[13] Circulating B cell abnormalities in SLE patients include: increased proliferation, increased calcium flux, hyper-responsiveness to physiologic stimuli, and altered production of and response to cytokines.[2] See Table 2.2, Cytokines and chemokines in lupus.

Table 2.2 Cytokines, chemokines, and interferons

Cytokine/chemokine	Actions	Role in SLE
Interferon α/β/ω	Dendritic cell maturation, Ig class switching, induction of immunoregulatory molecules	Increase serum levels in active disease Target for future therapy
Tumour necrosis factor-α	More research need in the role of SLE	Increased serum levels
IL-1	Pro-inflammatory	Increased serum levels in active disease
IL-2	Activation induced cell death of helper T cells and generation of Tregs	Decreased serum levels
IL-4		Increased serum levels
IL-6	Promotes terminal B cell differentiation to plasma cells, augmentation of immunoglobulins, synthesis of acute phase reactants, osteoclastic differentiation	Increased serum levels correlate with disease activity Target for future therapy
IL-10	Pro-inflammatory: augments B cell proliferation and promotes Ig class switching Anti-inflammatory: inhibits T cell activation and TNF-α secretion	Increased serum levels
IL-12	Promotes expansion of helper T1 cells and natural killer cells	Increased serum levels
IL-17	Pro-inflammatory, stimulates B lymphocytes	Found in target tissues of SLE patients, increased levels correlate with disease activity Target for future therapy
IL-18	Promotes expansion of helper T1 cells and natural killer cells	Increased in serum levels
Transforming growth factor-β	Down-regulates autoimmune responses	Decreased in SLE
BAFF/BLyS	Promotes B cell survival, Ig class switching, up-regulates cytokine production and co-stimulatory molecules on dendritic cells	Increased serum levels in active disease Target for belimumab
IL-8/IP-10/MCP-1/ Fractaline	Recruits inflammatory cells to sites of organ inflammation	Increased in renal tissue of lupus nephritis and serum of lupus nephritis
TWEAK(TNF-like weak inducer of apoptosis)		Elevations in urine have 50% sensitivity and 90% specificity for active glomerulonephritis
Neutrophil gelatinase associated lipocalin	Promotes apoptosis	Increased in urine during active lupus nephritis
Chemokine C-X-C motif ligand 16f	Recruits T cells and natural killer cells to tissues	Increased in urine during active lupus nephritis

Abbreviations: BAFF: B cell activating factor; ByLS: B lymphocyte stimulator inhibitor; IL: interleukin; IP: interferon-gamma inducible protein; MCP-1: monocyte chemoattractant protein-1; TNF: tumour necrosis factor.

Genetics and epigenetics in SLE

Genetic predisposition to SLE is an important factor in the development of disease. While certain gene polymorphisms carry a higher association with disease than others, in the vast majority of patients there is no single 'lupus gene'. Rather, patients inherit multiple high-risk alleles, which, in the setting of epigenetic phenomena and environmental triggers, result in the manifestation of clinical symptoms. Twin studies highlight the importance of genetics in the development of lupus. Monozygotic twins have a 10-fold higher risk of disease than dizygotic twins, and siblings of lupus patients have a 8–20-fold higher risk of developing disease when compared with the general population.[2] However, concordance for disease in monozygotic twins is only 24–58%, highlighting the environmental influences and multifactorial nature of the disease.[16]

There are certain gene mutations that confer much greater risk of disease development than others—but they are rare. These include homozygous deficiencies of C1q, an early complement component; mutations of TREX1 and DNASE1, which regulate DNA breakdown; and ACP5 and SPP1 polymorphisms, which cause increased activity of interferon alpha.[2] Genome wide association studies (GWAS) have identified over 50 gene loci associated with the development of lupus.[16] However, only a few of these genetic variants confer very high risk for SLE when inherited alone. For example, 93% of patients with a deficiency of C1q, which is responsible for clearance of IC and apoptotic cells, will develop a lupus-like syndrome. Approximately 75% of patients with a C4a and b deficiency develop glomerulonephritis. These patients often have glomerulonephritis, CNS, and skin disease. Other complement deficiencies carry a lower, but significant risk of disease. A missense mutation in TREX 1, which is responsible for DNA degradation, has been implicated in neuropsychiatric lupus, with 25% of patients with the mutation developing disease.[2]

The majority of patients inherit several gene polymorphisms. Each individual mutation carries only a modest odds ratio, but together they are associated with development of disease and increased disease activity. The majority of these genetic variants are single nucleotide polymorphisms, though deletions and low copy number variants also play a role.[2] Genetic mutations associated with SLE affect many important pathways in the immune system, including the innate and adaptive immune responses as well as IC clearance. The most common site of predisposing genetic alleles in SLE is found within the major histocompatibility complex (MHC). Also known as the human leucocyte antigen (HLA) region, it is divided into three smaller regions. Regions I and II encode the well-known HLA genes (HLA-A, -B, -C, -DR, -DQ and -DP), which play a role in antigen presentation to T cells, while region III encodes for early complement components, (C2, C4, factor B), cytokines such as TNF-α, and heat shock proteins. Up to 75% of patients with SLE (from all ethnicities) have at least one predisposing HLA gene polymorphism. Polymorphisms within HLA-DR2 and -DR3 are strongly associated with disease in white Europeans and European Americans. Heterozygotes with one of these mutations have 1.2 to 1.5 times the risk of disease, while risk in a homozygote with a DR2 or DR3 polymorphism is 1.8 to 2.8 times higher compared with wild-type carriers. Polymorphisms in other disease-associated genes including IRF7, TLR7/8, TNFS4 and IL10, have been seen in patients of African American, Asian, Mexican, and European decent.[2] Predisposing genes encoding for proteins in innate immune pathways include those involved with toll-like receptor pathways, interferon signalling, and nuclear factor-kappaB (NF-βB) signalling. These mutations ultimately lead to the enhanced interferon alpha signature that is characteristic of SLE. One high-risk allele of the STAT gene (signal transducer and activator of transcription gene), rs7574866, is associated with particularly aggressive disease with high titre anti-dsDNA, younger age at onset of disease, and increased risk of nephritis.[2] Significant tissue damage develops in SLE patients as a result of dysfunctional IC clearance. Gene polymorphisms associated with SLE have been discovered among genes encoding for complement components, phagocytosis, and DNA degradation. These include the aforementioned mutations, TREX1 and C1q.[2]

The adaptive immune system guards against foreign pathogens via cytotoxic killing and protective antibody production. Loss of T cell and B cell tolerance leads to the development of autoAb, which persist in SLE but are down-regulated in normal immune systems. Mutations in genes encoding for tolerance pathways, as well as those that dictate increased B and T cell signalling have been implicated in the development of SLE.[16] Polymorphisms in the gene for IL-10, a regulatory cytokine important in B cell activation and T cell inhibition, confers risk for SLE in large population genome-wide association studies.[2] A diagram of several known gene polymorphisms and the immunologic pathways with which they are associated is shown in Figure 2.2.

Genome level polymorphisms, deletions, and gene interactions account for <50% of susceptibility to SLE. Epigenetics, the inheritable transcriptional potential of a cell to translate nucleotide sequences into messenger RNA and functional proteins, plays an important role in the pathogenesis of lupus.[2] DNA within the cell is very precisely packaged within the nucleus. DNA strands are wound around a core of histone proteins forming nucleosomes, which are arranged into a tightly bound formation known as chromatin. In order for transcription units to bind DNA and synthesize mRNA and proteins, they must have access to the genes. In healthy cells, the chromatin is arranged in such a way that necessary genes are found on open sections of chromatin, while those genes that are unnecessary or detrimental to cell function are packed tightly

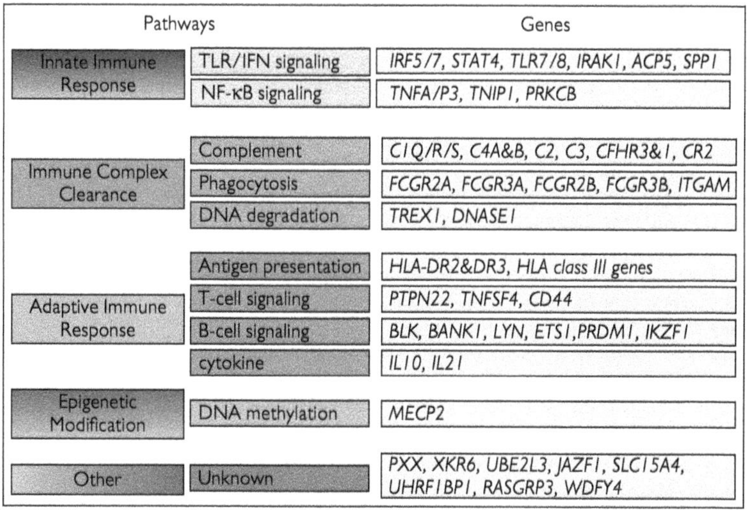

Pathways		Genes
Innate Immune Response	TLR/IFN signaling	IRF5/7, STAT4, TLR7/8, IRAK1, ACP5, SPP1
	NF-κB signaling	TNFA/P3, TNIP1, PRKCB
Immune Complex Clearance	Complement	C1Q/R/S, C4A&B, C2, C3, CFHR3&1, CR2
	Phagocytosis	FCGR2A, FCGR3A, FCGR2B, FCGR3B, ITGAM
	DNA degradation	TREX1, DNASE1
Adaptive Immune Response	Antigen presentation	HLA-DR2&DR3, HLA class III genes
	T-cell signaling	PTPN22, TNFSF4, CD44
	B-cell signaling	BLK, BANK1, LYN, ETS1,PRDM1, IKZF1
	cytokine	IL10, IL21
Epigenetic Modification	DNA methylation	MECP2
Other	Unknown	PXX, XKR6, UBE2L3, JAZF1, SLC15A4, UHRF1BP1, RASGRP3, WDFY4

Figure 2.2 Important immunologic pathways in the pathogenesis of SLE as highlighted by the identified susceptibility genes.

Abbreviations: IFN, interferon; NF-κB, nuclear factor kappa B; TLR, toll-like receptor: Reprinted from Dubois' Lupus Erythematosus and Related Syndromes, 8th Edition, Wallace and Hahn, Chapter 4: Genetics of Human SLE; Deng and Tsao, copyright (2013) with permission from Elsevier.

away, thereby preventing binding of transcription units.[2] Epigenetic modifications, which direct the folding and unfolding of DNA, alter the availability of gene expression at each level of organization. Modifications include methylation of the DNA itself, histone acetylation, ubiquination, and phosphorylation, as well as binding of micro-RNAs to transcriptional regions.[16] These changes lead to defects in gene transcription, post-translational regulation, messenger RNA editing, alternative splicing, and protein modification.[2] Epigenetic changes in DNA methylation may occur as a result of aging, or in response to certain environmental factors such as UV light, drugs, and diet. Methylation changes are regulated by DNA methyltransferases. SLE patients are known to have hypomethylated DNA in T cells compared with healthy controls, resulting in expression of altered cell-surface protein patterns and auto-reactive T cells. Likewise, changes in histone configuration and winding of DNA within the nucleosomes have been associated with SLE.[2]

MicroRNAs (miRNAs) also alter gene expression, but do so at the post-transcriptional level. These non-coding RNAs function to down-regulate gene expression. MicroRNA binding sites are found throughout the genome, but are in especially high concentrations within the mRNA products of immune function genes.[2] Many groups have identified specific miRNAs associated with SLE; a few of those confirmed in different cohorts include miR-155, which regulates both the innate and adaptive immune response; miR-182, which decreases synthesis of IL-2 by blocking Foxo1; and miR-146a, which activates the production of interferon-alpha.[2]

Environmental triggers in SLE

Environmental factors impact the development of SLE in several ways, including induction of apoptosis, of immune reactivity, and production of autoAb via breakdown of immune tolerance.[2] Exposure to ultraviolet light, especially UVB, is the best known and most understood trigger for disease activity. UV light triggers apoptosis of keratinocytes, thereby increasing the quantity of self-antigen presented to the immune system. UVB light also alters the structure of DNA in the dermis, rendering it more immunogenic.[2] Certain infections, including those in the Epstein–Barr virus family, have been implicated in triggering and exacerbating SLE. One mechanism by which this is thought to occur is molecular mimicry, where the Epstein–Barr nuclear antigen 1 is similar to the Ro/SSA particle, inducing enhanced immune response to self-antigens.[2] Many patients with SLE develop a flare in the setting of viral and bacterial infections. Silica dust, found in many common construction materials including cement, brick, and drywall, has been associated with the onset of SLE in certain individuals, especially those with higher risk occupations.[17,18]

UV light, infections and silica dust are all known to induce oxidative stress, an important factor in the development of tissue disease in SLE. Cigarette smoke, air pollution, and exposure to elemental mercury are other important inducers of oxidative stress, and exposure to these toxins has been associated with an increased odds ratio of disease in certain SLE populations versus healthy controls.[19] Drug-induced lupus is a well-known disease process, in which individuals develop a lupus-like syndrome after exposure to a host of drugs including procainamide, interferons, TNF inhibitors, anticonvulsants, minocycline, lithium, and hydralazine.[19] Certain drugs induce epigenetic changes within DNA in T cells by lowering the level of DNA methyltransferase 1 (Dnmt1). Disruption in DNA methylation alters gene expression in T cells and converts a healthy immune response into an auto-reactive cascade.[15] Withdrawal of these drugs usually results in resolution of disease. Some studies have also proposed that a methyl-poor diet may be correlated with the development and flare of SLE in genetically predisposed patients.[19]

The interaction of genes, environmental factors, and the epigenetic modifications that these factors produce, highlights the complexity of this disease and offers opportunities for further research into the pathogenesis of disease.

Role of gender

SLE has a marked female predilection; in child-bearing years the female to male ratio is 9:1. In prepubertal and postmenopausal age groups, the ratio is 3:1. Increased risk in females is probably related to sex hormone levels (particularly oestradiol), epigenetic changes, environmental exposures, and risk alleles on the X chromosome. Healthy women exposed to oestrogen-containing hormone replacement therapies or oral contraceptives have a small but significantly increased risk for developing SLE. Oestradiol and related hormones have multiple effects on the immune system; a major effect is allowing autoreactive B cells at certain developmental stages to escape deletion, thus promoting breaks in immune tolerance and permitting survival of autoreactive B cells. Children and men with SLE in general have inherited more susceptibility alleles for SLE than the at-higher-risk women of child-bearing age. The Trex1 gene (mutations in which increase the risk for SLE), is located on the X chromosome (see discussion of 'Genetics and epigenetics in SLE' in this chapter). With regard to epigenetics, the suppressed X chromosome in women is more highly methylated than the expressed X; the methylated DNA can be antigenic. Finally, it may be that women are exposed more than men to certain environmental stimuli, such as silica-containing soap powders.[17,18]

References

1. Cozzani E, Drosera M, Gasparini G, Parodi A. Serology of lupus erythematosus: Correlation between immunopathological features and clinical aspects. *Autoimmune diseases* doi: 10.1155/2014/321359. Epub 6 Feb 2014.

2. Hahn BH, Wallace DJ (Eds). *Dubois' lupus erythematosus and related syndromes* 8th Ed.: Elsevier Saunders, Philidelphia; 2013.

3. Pisetsky DS. Standardization of anti-DNA antibody assays. *Immunologic research* 2013;56: 420–4.

4. Friedman DM, Rupel A, Buyon JP. Epidemiology, etiology, detection, and treatment of autoantibody-associated congenital heart block in neonatal lupus. *Current rheumatology reports* 2007;9:101–8.

5. Shi ZR, Cao CX, Tan GZ, Wang L. The association of serum anti-ribosomal P antibody with clinical and serological disorders in systemic lupus erythematosus: a systematic review and meta-analysis. *Lupus* doi: 10.1177/0961203314560003. Epub 17 Nov 2014.

6. Leffler J, Bengtsson AA, Blom AM. The complement system in systemic lupus erythematosus: an update. *Ann Rheum Dis* 2014;73:1601–6.

7. Ahmadpoor P, Dalili N, Rostami M. An update on pathogenesis of systemic lupus erythematosus. *Iranian journal of kidney diseases* 2014;8:171–84.

8. Aringer M, Gunther C, Lee-Kirsch MA. Innate immune processes in lupus erythematosus. *Clin Immunol* 2013;147:216–22.

9. Kaplan MJ, Radic M. Neutrophil extracellular traps: double-edged swords of innate immunity. *J Immunol* 2012;189:2689–95.

10. Munoz LE, Janko C, Schulze C, et al. Autoimmunity and chronic inflammation: two clearance-related steps in the etiopathogenesis of SLE. *Autoimmunity reviews* 2010;10:38–42.

11. Sahu R, Bethunaickan R, Singh S, Davidson A. Structure and function of renal macrophages and dendritic cells from lupus-prone mice. *Arthritis Rheumatol* (Hoboken, NJ) 2014;66:1596–607.

12. Mak A, Kow NY. The pathology of T cells in systemic lupus erythematosus. *J Immunol Res* doi: 10.1155/2014/419029. Epub 23 Apr 2014.

13. Sang A, Zheng YY, Morel L. Contributions of B cells to lupus pathogenesis. *Mol Immunol* 2014;62:329–38.

14. Tsokos GC. Systemic lupus erythematosus. *N Engl J Med* 2011;365:2110–21.

15. Martin JC, Baeten DL, Josien R. Emerging role of IL-17 and Th17 cells in systemic lupus erythematosus. *Clin Immunol* 2014;154:1–12.

16. Deng Y, Tsao BP. Advances in lupus genetics and epigenetics. *Curr Opin Rheumatol* 2014;26:482–92.

17. Finckh A, Cooper GS, Chibnik LB, et al. Occupational silica and solvent exposures and risk of systemic lupus erythematosus in urban women. *Arthritis Rheum* 2006;54:3648–54.

18. Costenbader KH, Gay S, Alarcon-Riquelme ME, Iaccarino L, Doria A. Genes, epigenetic regulation and environmental factors: which is the most relevant in developing autoimmune diseases? *Autoimmun Rev* 2012;11:604–9.

19. Somers EC, Richardson BC. Environmental exposures, epigenetic changes and the risk of lupus. *Lupus* 2014;23:568–76.

Chapter 3

Epidemiology of systemic lupus erythematosus

Caroline Gordon and S. Sam Lim

Key points

- Lupus occurs worldwide and is most common in women and people of African, Hispanic, and Asian (especially Chinese) descent.
- There is also a high incidence and prevalence in First Nation Canadians, American Indians, Alaska Natives, and Australian Aborigines compared with people of white North European origin.
- Renal disease is more common and is associated with a worse prognosis in all of these ethnic minorities, and lupus often presents at a younger age in these groups than those of white North European origin.
- Although survival rates have improved over the last 60 years, mortality rates are still increased as indicated by standardized mortality ratios of 2.0–3.0 compared with age- and sex-matched local populations in recent studies.
- Patients with a history of active severe lupus are most likely to develop damage and to die prematurely, predominantly from renal disease, infection, and cardiovascular disease.
- Management of lupus needs to be targeted at reducing factors that increase the risk of lupus disease activity, damage, and mortality.

Introduction

Systemic lupus erythematosus is more common than many people realize, especially in certain racial and ethnic groups. This chapter reviews the worldwide frequency and distribution of lupus and discusses the factors associated with increased incidence and prevalence in certain populations. The outcomes for these patients are also disparate, but premature death remains a significant challenge for physicians caring for these patients despite improving survival rates over the last 60 years. Risk factors for poor outcomes will be discussed, particularly those that should be amenable to change.

The nature of the studies reported in the literature is varied, and it should be noted that there are many biases that may influence the reported data due to varying methods of case ascertainment; different definitions used; and the population base for the study, which may reflect specific types of healthcare provision. There are very few community-based population studies collecting data on all lupus patients using a defined disease classification in a specific geographical area over a finite time period, which makes reliable comparisons between studies difficult. Nevertheless certain conclusions can be drawn from the rapidly increasing literature about the epidemiology of lupus and this will be summarized in this chapter.

Incidence and prevalence

In general the studies from North America and Europe are of better quality in terms of study design than those from South America, Africa, Asia, and Australia. The incidence and prevalence rates vary with the nature of the population studied, given the important influence of age, gender, and racial/ethnic background on disease development due to the interplay of genetic and environmental factors. Data on incidence and prevalence worldwide are summarized in Figures 3.1 (colour version on inside cover) and 3.2 (colour version on inside cover) and Tables 3.1–3.5. It should be remembered that there may be under-reporting of cases where access to health care is limited or for mild disease, unless mechanisms are in place to capture patients attending a variety of healthcare providers.

In the USA the most recent population-based studies in Georgia and Michigan found the incidence to be close to 5.5/100,000/year and the prevalence to be 73/100,000. Incidence rates in the USA of about 4.5 (range 2.0–7.6) and prevalence rates between 19 and 159 had been reported previously and were dependent on: how lupus was defined; what and how many methods of case ascertainment and age standardization were used; and the ethnic and racial background of the population.

European studies have shown similar variation in the incidence and prevalence rates, depending on the population studied and the study design, with incidence rates between 1.0 and 4.9/100,000/year and prevalence rates from 28.0 to 97.0/100,000. The most recent study from the UK by Rees et al. covering 1999–2012 using the Clinical Practice Research Datalink (CPRD), previously known as the General Practice Research Database (GPRD), suggested that the incidence was falling and the prevalence in the UK was rising compared with previous studies using this database. However, it should be noted that this study did not validate cases and did not use any validated classification criteria for lupus, although they did present three alternative case definitions, only one of which required supporting evidence in the medical record. The latter method suggested an incidence 4.6/100,000 and a point prevalence in 2012 of 88.1/100,000. This study analysed patients with diagnoses recorded in general practice using Read codes, a coded system of recording clinical terms used in the National Health Service in the UK. The authors may have over-estimated lupus disease in some areas because patients did not have to meet specific classification criteria for lupus, and due to the lack of Read codes for patients with incomplete criteria/undifferentiated connective tissue disease, these were not distinguished from those with systemic lupus erythematosus. However, they are likely to have missed cases from the ethnic minorities living in areas where few general practitioners (GPs) contribute to the database such as the West Midlands, which has a significant Afro-Caribbean and South Asian population that are known to have high rates of lupus from previous studies (Johnson et al. 1995). In the GPRD study they reported a lower incidence in the West Midlands (3.9/100,000) than in the white-dominated East of England (6.0/100,000).

The effect of gender and age on incidence and prevalence

Lupus is about 10 times more common in females than males, particularly during the reproductive years. The gender difference is much smaller under the age of 10, when the disease is rare and over the age of 60 years. For example, age-adjusted incidence

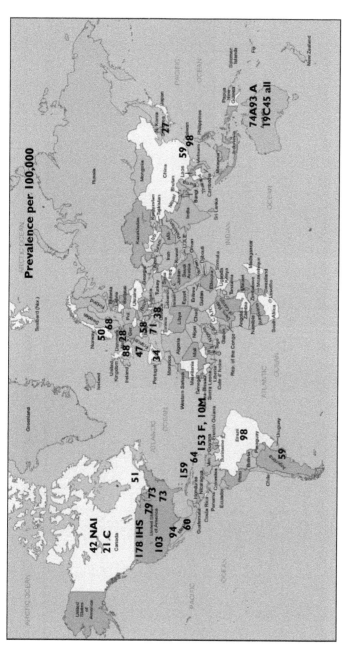

Figure 3.1 World map showing the incidence of lupus in different countries per 100,000 population per year. (See colour version on inside cover.)

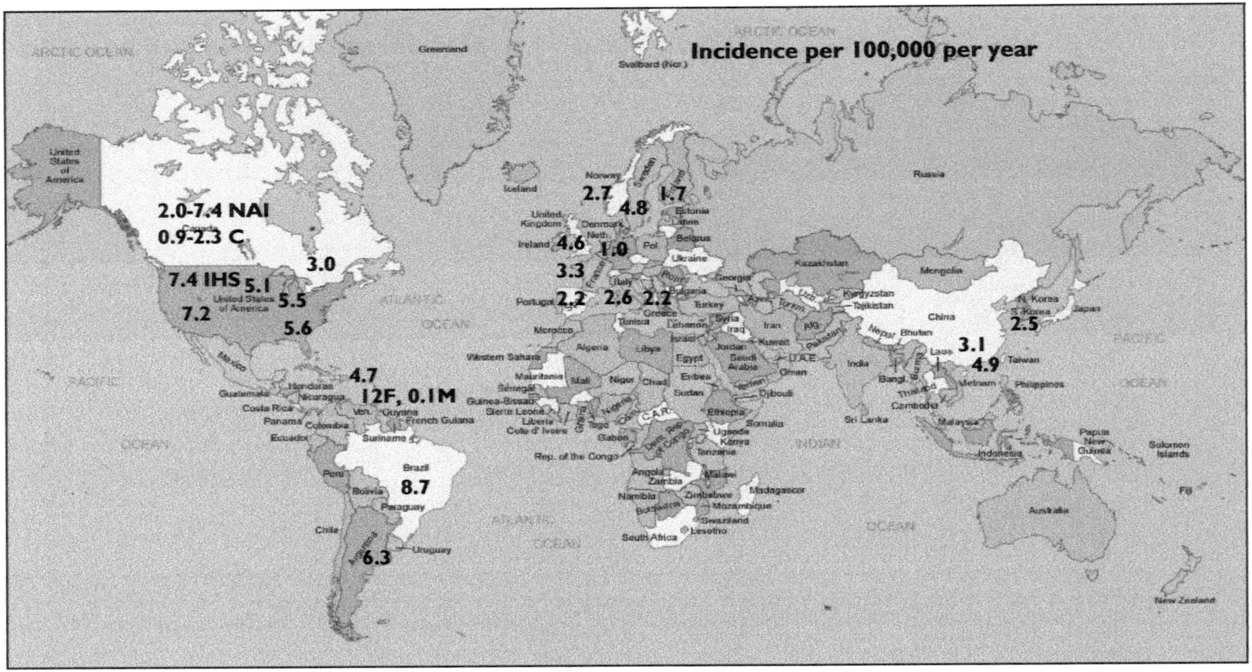

Figure 3.2 World map showing the prevalence of lupus in different countries per 100,000 population. (See colour version on inside cover.)

Table 3.1 Population-based studies of incidence and prevalence of SLE in North America, including the Caribbean and Puerto Rico

First author, year (ref)	Study location/country	Study years	Population at risk (race)	Incidence*	Prevalence**
Nossent 1992	Island of Curacao/ The Netherlands Antilles	1980–1990	146,500 (~95% African Caribbean, <5% white)	4.6 (overall) 7.9 (females) 1.1 (males)	48 (overall) 84 (female) 9 (male)
McCarty 1995	Allegheny County, PA/US	1985–1990	1,336,449 (All races)	2.4 (overall)	ND
Uramoto 1999	Rochester, MN/US	1950–1992	Rochester population (white)	3.1+ (overall) 5.6*(1980–1992) 1.5*(1950–1979)	122* (Jan 1992)
Peschken 2000	Province of Manitoba/ Canada	1980–1996	~1,100,000 (NAI and NI)	2.0–7.4 (NAI) 0.9–2.3 (NI)	42.3 (NAI) 20.6 (NI)
Walsh 2001	Nogales, AZ/US	1997	19,489 (92% Mexican American)	ND	94 (overall)
Deligny 2002	Martinique Island/French West Indies	1990–1999	381,427 (Mostly African Caribbean)	4.7 (overall)	64.2 (overall)
Ward 2004	NHANES III (sample of US population)	2000	20,050 (All races)	ND	241 (self-report) 54 (on SLE drugs)
Naleway 2005	Rural area North Central Wisconsin/US	1991–2001	77,280 (97% white)	5.1* (definite) 8.2* (definite females) 1.9* (definite males)	79* (definite) 132* (definite female) 25* (definite male)
Molina 2007	Puerto Rico/US	2003	552,733 private insured people (Race ND)	ND	159 (overall) 277 (female) 25 (male)

(continued)

Table 3.1 Continued

First author, year (ref)	Study location/country	Study years	Population at risk (race)	Incidence*	Prevalence**
Bernatsky 2007	Quebec/Canada	1994–2003	~7.5 million (All races)	3.0 (PB) 2.8 (HDD)	33 (PB) 33 (HDD) 51 (composite) 45 (Bayesian model)
Pelaez-Ballestas 2011	Mexico City, Nuevo Leon, Yucatan, Sinaloa, Chihuahua/ Mexico	2008–2010 depending on region	Sample of 19,213 people age 18 and above (Race ND)	ND	60^(overall) 80 (female) 40 (male) 90 (Mexico City) 40 (N Leon) 70 (Yucatan) 40 (Sinaloa) 40 (Chihuahua)
Flower 2012	Nationwide/ Barbados	2000–2009	268,792 (2000, 93% African origin, 3% white, 3% mixed)	12.21 (women) 0.84 (men)	Point prevalence: 152.6 (women) 10.1 (men)
Lim 2014	Fulton and DeKalb counties of Atlanta, Georgia/US	2002–2004	1,552,970	5.6	73
Somers 2014	Wayne and Washtenaw counties, Michigan/US	2002–2004	2.4 million	5.5	72.8
Ferucci 2014	Indian Health Service/US	2007–2009	211,916 (2007, American Indian/Alaska Native)	7.4	178
Furst 2013	US managed care	2003–2008	1557 Age >18	7.2	81.1 in 2003 102.9 in 2008

*Per 100,000 per year; **per 100,000; ^age adjusted to national or regional population; °age and sex adjusted.

Abbreviations: ACR: American College of Rheumatism; DB: database; GP: general practitioners; HDD: hospital discharge data; MR: medical record; NA: not available; NAI: North American Indian; ND: not determined; NI: non Indian; PB: physician billing.

Table 3.2 Population-based studies of incidence and prevalence of SLE in South America

First author, year (ref)	Study location/ country	Study years	Population at risk (race)	Incidence*	Prevalence**
Vilar 2002	Natal city, Rio Grande do Norte/Brazil	2000	493,239 people aged >15 (Race ND)	8.7^ (overall) 14.1 (females) 2.2 (males)	ND
Senna 2004	Montes Claros, Minas Gerais/Brazil	ND	Sample of 3038 people age >16 years (38% white, 62% non-white)	ND	98 (overall) 90 (male) 110 (female)
Scolnick 2014	Buenos Aires/ Argentina	1998–2009	127,959 aged >18	6.3 8.9 women 2.6 men	58.6 83.2 women 23 men

*Per 100,000 per year, **per 100,000; ^sex-adjusted.
Abbreviations: ND: not determined.

Table 3.3 Population-based studies of incidence and prevalence of SLE in Asia

First author, year (ref)	Study location/ country	Study years	Population at risk (race)	Incidence*	Prevalence**
Huang 2004	Nationwide/ Taiwan	1999	5.78 million children aged <16	ND	6.3 (overall) 11.2 (girls) 1.8 (boys)
Mok 2003	Hong Kong/ China	2001	1.49 million (Hong Kong Chinese)	ND	58.8
Mok 2008	Hong Kong/ China	2000–2006	1 million (Hong Kong Chinese)	3.1 (2000) 2.8 (2006)	ND
Chiu 2010	Nationwide/ Taiwan	2000–2007	22.28 million (in 2000) 22.96 million (in 2007)	8.1 (2001–2007)	42.2 (2000) 67.4 (2007)
Shim 2014	Nationwide/ S. Korea	2006–2010	~50 million	2.5	20.6 (2006) 26.5 (2010)
Ju 2014	Nationwide/ S. Korea	2004–2006		ND	18.8–21.7
See 2013	Taiwan	2005–2009	1 million	7.2	
Yeh 2013	Taiwan	2003–2008	96% population of Taiwan	4.87	97.5

Table 3.4 Population-based studies of incidence and prevalence of SLE in Australia

First author, year (ref)	Study location/ country	Study years	Population at risk (race)	Incidence*	Prevalence**
Bossingham 2003	Far North Queensland/ Australia	1996–1998	238,000 (mostly Caucasian, 11.8% Aboriginal)	ND	45.3 (overall) 92.8 (Aborigines)
Segasothy 2001	Alice Springs and Barkly regions/ Australia	1990–1999	19,000 Aborigine 31,000 Caucasian	ND	73.5 Aborigine 19.3 Caucasian

rates in Georgia were recently reported to be five times higher among women than men (9.2/100,000/year vs 1.8/100,000/year) and age-adjusted prevalence rates were nearly nine times higher in women than in men (127.6 vs 14.7 per 100,000). The data from Michigan using very similar methods over the same time interval (2002–2004) was almost identical (female incidence 9.3/10,000/year and prevalence 128.7/100,000). The incidence was more than six times higher and the prevalence was ten times higher in females than males. Similar results were found in the recent UK GPRD study where the female incidence was six times higher (7.8/100,000/year vs 1.3/100,000/ year in males) and the female prevalence was seven times higher (152.5/100,000 vs 22.2/100,000 in males).

The mean age (standard deviation (SD)) at diagnosis in the US population-based studies with multiple methods of case ascertainment was similar in females and males (39.3 years (SD 16.6) in Michigan and 40.5 years (SD 16.5) in Georgia). Incidence and prevalence rates increased with age during the reproductive years in females but were fairly constant in males. In the UK GPRD study with a predominantly white population, the mean age at diagnosis was older at 48.9 years (SD 16.9) and more comparable to previous and recent North European studies suggesting lupus is most likely to develop in the 40–59 age group. Women in the UK study were significantly younger than men at diagnosis: 48.3 years (SD 16.8) versus 52.1 years (SD 17.2) (p <0.001).

The incidence and prevalence of paediatric lupus has been hard to determine as studies vary in the age groups studied, definitions used, and completeness of populations studied. In the recent US study in Georgia, with 399 incident cases meeting revised ACR classification criteria, there were 24 incident cases in females <20 years old, of which only five were under 12 years old. In 2012, Hiraki et al. published a specific study on paediatric lupus among children enrolled in Medicaid in the US. There were 2959 cases out of 30,420,597, giving a prevalence of SLE of 9.7/100,000 and the average annual incidence was 2.2/100,000. Rates of SLE were higher in girls than boys and in non-white racial/ethnic groups, as had been reported from other countries including the UK, Australia, and Taiwan. In the UK paediatric study published in 2012 by Watson et al., the female to male ratio was 5.6:1, and males were younger than females at diagnosis. In a recent study from Finland, the incidence in white children was low, at 0.39 per 100,000.

The effect of race and ethnicity on incidence and prevalence

Lupus is more common in people of African origin that have migrated to North America or Europe than those of white North European origin. Women of African origin have some of the highest incidence and prevalence rates reported worldwide

Table 3.5 Population-based studies of incidence and prevalence of SLE in Europe

First author, year (ref)	Study location/country	Study years	Population at risk (race)	Annual incidence*	Prevalence**
Hopkinson 1994	Nottingham/ UK	1989–1990	601,693 (all races)	4.0[+] (overall) 3.4[+] (white) 31.9[+] (black) 4.1[+] (Asian) ND (Chinese)	24.7[+](overall) 20.3[+] (white) 207.0[+] (black) 48.8[+] (Asian) 92.9[+] (Chinese)
Johnson 1995	Birmingham and Solihull Districts/ UK	1991–1992	872,877 (all races)	3.8^ (overall)	27.7^ (overall) 20.7^ (white) 111.8^ (black) 46.7^ (Asian)
Voss 1998	Funen County/ Denmark	1980–1994	387,841 (white)	1.0 (1980) 3.6 (1994)	22.2[+] (definite) 5.2 (incomplete)
Stahl-Hallengren 2000	Lund and Orup Districts/ South Sweden	1986–1991	174,952 (mostly white)	4.8(1987–1991) 4.5 if patients with >4 ACR are assessed	42.0 (1986) 68.0 (1991)
Nossent 2001	Finnmark and Troms counties/ Norway	1978–1996	224,403 (mostly white)	2.9^ (overall) 2.4 (1978–1986) 2.7 (1987–1995)	49.7^ (1996)
Lopez 2003	Asturias/ Northern Spain	1998–2002	1,073,971 (mostly white)	2.15 (overall)	34.1 (2002)
Alamanos 2003	6 districts of northwest Greece	1982–2001	488,435	1.41^ (1982–1986) 1.95^ (1987–1991) 2.19^ (1997–2001)	38.12^ (2001)
Benucci 2005	Scandicci-Le Signe(Florence)/Italy	2002	71,204 (>18 years old)	ND	71

(continued)

Table 3.5 Continued

First author, year (ref)	Study location/country	Study years	Population at risk (race)	Annual incidence*	Prevalence**
Govoni 2006	Ferrara District/Italy	1996–2002	~346,000 (mostly white)	2.01 (2000) 1.15 (2001) 2.60 (2002)	57.9 (overall)
Nightingale 2006 and 2007	Nationwide/UK	1992–1998	12,911,216 person-years (all races)	3.0 (overall)	25.0 (1992) 40.7 (1998)
Somers 2007	Nationwide/UK	1990–1999	33,666,320 person-years (all races)	4.7+ (overall)	ND
Laustrup 2009	Funen County/ Denmark	1995–2003	386,884 (mostly white, ≥15 years old)	1.04 (definite) 0.36 (incomplete)	28.3 (definite) 7.53 (incomplete)
Anagnostopoulos 2010	Prefecture of Magnesia/ Greece	2007–2008	176,433	ND	110
Simard 2014	Nationwide./ Sweden	2010	9,340,682	ND	46–85
Rees 2014	Nationwide sample/ UK	1999–2012	~12 million	4.91	64.99 (1999) 97.04 (2012)
Arnaud 2014	Nationwide sample/ France	2010	~58.2 million (race/ethnicity unavailable)	3.32	47
Elfving 2014	Nationwide	2000–2007		1.69 Sex ratio 6.43 Highest age 40–59 years Children incidence 0.39	-

*Per 100,000 per year; **Per 100,000; +Age standardized to national or regional population; +Age standardized to European population.

Abbreviations: CPRD: Clinical Practice Research Datalink; CTD: connective tissue disease; GP: general practitioners; HDD: hospital discharge data; MR: medical record; ND: not determined; UK: United Kingdom.

and they usually develop lupus at a younger age and have a higher risk of lupus nephritis and end-stage renal disease.

The US studies from Georgia and Michigan reported incidence rates 2–3 times higher in black women than white women (13.4 vs 4.7 in Georgia), with peak values in black women aged 20–29 years in Michigan and 30–39 years in Georgia. The incidence in men was four times higher in black men than white men in Georgia (3.2 vs 0.7) with no significant differences with age in either racial group, but absolute numbers were small. In the recent UK study, incidence was over four times higher in people of Black Caribbean origin compared with those of white background in the GP practices where this could be assessed.

In these recent US studies, black women had very high prevalence rates compared with white women (196.2/100,000 vs 59.0/100,000 in Georgia, and 186.3/100,000 vs 86.7/100,000 in Michigan). Thus lupus affected about 1 in 500 black women as reported previously for Afro-Caribbean women in the UK. Prevalence in females from Barbados was reported recently to be 153/100,000 versus 10/100,000 in Afro-Caribbean males.

Other groups with a high prevalence of lupus include American Indians and Alaska Natives (178/100,000), as do Aborigines from Australia (73.5–92.8/100,000). In one study from Taiwan published in 2013, Chinese patients were reported to have prevalence rates up to 97.5/100,000, but more recent studies from Korea in 2014 found lower rates (18.8 to 26.5/100,000).

Mortality

All studies addressing mortality and lupus have shown increased standardized mortality ratios (SMR, the ratio of observed to expected deaths which are sex and age-adjusted) of at least 2.0 compared with the relevant local population. The original reports on mortality in SLE in the 1950s suggested that only 50% of lupus patients survived 4 years. With earlier diagnosis, improved treatment, and monitoring of the disease and comorbidities, the survival rate has improved over the last 60 years. But it should be remembered that mortality has reduced in general, with figures of up to 70% reduction in mortality in the general population in the US between 1965 and 2005, largely due to a reduction in deaths from heart attacks and strokes.

In the 1980s 5-year survival rates in lupus patients of 64–87% were reported, but by 2008, figures of 92–98% were reported, especially in Europe and North America (see Table 3.6). By this time 10-year survival rates of 83–98%, 15-year survival rates of 76–85%, and 20-year survival rates of up to 77% were being reported in developed countries. The Toronto group followed 1241 patients for up to 36 years and published in 2008 that the overall SMR for 1970–2005, was estimated to be 4.53 (95% CI, 3.96–5.19) assuming that patients lost to follow-up were censored at last visit. They reported a reduction in SMR from 12.60 (95% CI, 9.13–17.39) for the first decade 1970–1979, down to 3.46 (95% CI, 2.71–4.40) for 1996 to 2005.

The largest lupus mortality study to date was published by the Systemic Lupus International Collaborating Clinics (SLICC) group in 2006, with data from over 9500 patients followed mostly from 1970 to 2001 in 23 centres distributed over seven countries (Canada, USA, England, Scotland, Iceland, Sweden, Korea). This reported that the SMR was 2.4 for all lupus patients in this international study. However the SMRs in some countries, such as South Africa, remain lower with 5-year survival rates of only 58% in the late 2000s. As discussed further in the section on 'Race and ethnicity' later in

Table 3.6 Cumulative survival rates in studies published 2003–2014

Author	Year*	Study location	Comments	5-year survival (%)	10-year survival (%)	15-year survival (%)	20-year survival (%)
Cervera	2003	Europe		95	92	–	–
Mok	2005	China		92	83	80	–
Doria	2006	Italy		96	93	76	–
Kasitanon	2006	USA		95	91	85	78
Heller	2007	Saudi Arabia		92	–	–	–
Wadee	2007	S. Africa		58	–	–	–
Fanauchi	2007	Japan		94	92	–	77
Al-Saleh	2008	United Arab Emirates		94	–	–	–
Sun	2008	China		98	98	–	–
Al Arfaj	2009	Saudi Arabia		98	97	–	–
Eilertsen	2009	Norway		95	92	–	–
Rabbani	2009	Pakistan		80	77	75	75
Nossent	2010	Europe	14 countries	97	–	–	–
Kang	2011	Korea		98	–	–	–
Foocharoen	2011	Thailand		93	87	–	–
Flower	2012	Barbados	All Nephritis	80 68	–	–	–

	*Year	Country	Nephritis				
Yap	2012	China		99.5	98	–	91
Voss	2013	Denmark		94	87	73	–
Pamuk	2013	Turkey		96	92	89	–
Alonso	2014	Spain	Females	95	89	–	–
			Males	91	78**		
Merola	2014	US	<50 yrs^	99.5	98	–	–
			>50 yrs^	95	90		
Wu	2014	China	All	91	80	–	–
			Females	93	81		
			Males	82	62***		
Schmid	2014	Argentina	Private	91	–	–	–
			Public	78			
Elfving	2014	Finland	Females	95	–	–	–
			Males	88			
Lerang	2014	Sweden		95	90	–	–
Tavangar-Rad	2014	Iran		89	–	–	–

*Year published; **Survival in males not significantly different to females; ***Survival in males significantly worse than females; ^Age at diagnosis.

this chapter, certain racial/ethnic groups have not shown improvement in survival over the years and this affects SMRs observed in certain countries.

Recently a meta-analysis was published by Yurkovich in 2014, based on 12 studies reporting weighted-pooled summary estimates of SMRs (metaSMR) for all cause-cause and cause-specific mortality. The analysis included 27,210 patients enrolled between 1950 and 2008 (90% female). There were 4989 deaths in these lupus patients. The meta-SMR for all-cause mortality was 2.98 (95% CI, 2.32–3.83) suggesting that on average lupus patients are three times more likely to die than their peers of the same age and sex in the relevant local population.

The effect of gender on mortality

The SLICC mortality study found that the SMR for females was greater at 2.5 (95% CI, 2.3–2.7) than for males at 1.9 (95% CI, 1.7–2.2). Some studies have suggested that males have more severe lupus and a greater risk of dying than females with lupus, but these studies usually failed to compare mortality rates with the local population and/or may be the result of under-diagnosis of mild lupus in males. Using SMRs takes into consideration the fact that men tend to die at an earlier age than women. Lower sex and age-specific SMRs for men with SLE (4.0 with 95% CI, 2.9–5.4) compared with women (4.7 with 95% CI, 4.0–5.5) was reported in Toronto by Urowitz in 2008. Yurkovich reported no significant difference in the recent meta-analysis with a meta-SMR of 4.06 (95% CI, 3.11–5.30) in women and 3.41 (95% CI, 2.56–4.53) in men.

The effect of age on mortality

In 2002 the CDC reported that 36.4% of lupus patients dying were aged 15–44. Many studies, including the SLICC international mortality study with data up to 2001, have shown that the highest SMRs are seen in young patients with lupus, for whom the risk of dying would otherwise be very low. They published an SMR of 19.2 (95% CI, 14.7–24.7) for young adults aged 16–24; the SMR for all patients <40 years was 10.7 (95% CI, 9.5–11.9); and for those aged 40–59 the SMR was 3.7 (95% CI, 3.3–4.0). Even at older ages the SMR remains increased with those of 60 years and above having an SMR of 1.4 (95% CI, 1.3–1.5). More recent studies from Birmingham, UK have shown that there is still at least a five times higher risk of dying from lupus aged 20–24 than for that age in England and Wales overall, despite care in a dedicated lupus centre where patients have access to a national health service at all times.

There are still relatively few published studies on the outcomes of paediatric onset lupus, but given that the disease is often more severe in this group (see Chapter 8, Juvenile SLE) and often affects ethnic minorities more than whites, it is not surprising that studies have suggested higher mortality rates. For example in the LUpus in MInorities, NAture versus nurture (LUMINA) study, a multi-ethnic US lupus cohort, there was an almost two-fold higher mortality rate in juvenile onset as compared with adult onset lupus. Improved survival has been reported, as with adult onset lupus, over the years but there is considerable geographic variation. Thus developing countries still report much poorer outcomes than studies from North America and Europe.

The effect of race, ethnicity, geography, and socio-economic status on mortality

Walsh reported in 1995 that death rates in white females in the US were stable between the 1970s and 1991 at 4.6/million/year due to a reduction in deaths in those dying under age 45 and an increase in those dying over age 55. However between 1968 and 1991 deaths in African American women in the US were much higher and increased steadily by 30% to 18.7/million/year. Some of the higher death rate in African American women was due to the increased prevalence of lupus in these women, but the increased risk of death in this population has been confirmed in more recent studies assessing race-specific SMRs. However, data on racial stratification has not been available in most other countries until recently, although it has been widely recognized for over 50 years that black patients with lupus have a higher risk of dying than white patients, and there is increasing evidence that other ethnic minorities including people of Hispanic and Asian backgrounds, especially of Chinese origin, also have higher SMRs in various parts of the world. Comparison of death rates between countries is hampered by the small number of studies outside North America (US and Canada) and Europe (UK, Sweden, Denmark, Finland, Holland, Norway, Spain) although there is some data appearing from Malaysia, Singapore, India, China, Taiwan and South America including Chile and the Grupo Latinoamericano de Estudio del Lupus (GLADEL) collaboration.

The SLICC mortality study analysed data on race specific SMRs for US patients in their cohort and found that the risk of dying was nearly double in blacks/African Americans (SMR 2.6; 95% CI, 2.3–2.9) compared with whites/Caucasians (SMR 1.4; 95% CI, 1.2–1.7). There were no significant differences in the unadjusted SMR estimates based on geographic locations. The risk of dying was about twice that of the local population in all the countries studied with the lowest SMR in Sweden followed by Iceland, Scotland, US, Korea, England, and the highest SMR was in Canada but with considerable overlap of the 95% CI between all the countries.

In the LUMINA study published in 2007, 5-year survival rates were significantly lower for Texan Hispanics at 86.9% and African Americans at 89.8% than for Caucasians at 93.6% and Puerto Rican Hispanics at 97.2%. A multivariable Cox regression analysis found that disease activity damage, poverty, and older age significantly predicted mortality but not ethnicity.

The influence of racial/ethnic background is often confounded by the effects of social and economic status (SES) and there is increasing evidence that SES is a stronger predictor of mortality than racial/ethnic background. It was shown previously in the LUMINA study published in 2001 that the deaths were four times higher in those living on incomes below the US poverty level. Similar results have been observed in the GLADEL cohort. Poverty is often associated with poor education and reduced language skills; lack of access to medical care; poor social support; and poor compliance and non-adherence with treatment plans due to lack of understanding and difficulties attending appointments and/or paying for all aspects of medical care. Ward published in 2004 on the role of education and that even white lupus patients have twice the risk of dying if they have less than 8 years of education compared with those with more than 16 years of education.

The effects of associated low SES in many lupus patients of African, Hispanic, Chinese and other Asian descent plays a role in their increased risk of dying, with poor diet and poor housing contributing to the increased the risk of cardiovascular disease and infection seen in these patients. These risks are compounded by the consequences of not accessing medical care promptly and regularly, and reduced adherence to treatment which affects the outcome of these complications as well as the underlying lupus, especially as they often have renal disease. A study has shown that First Nation Canadians with lupus have an increased risk of deaths from all these causes, despite good theoretical access to health care, as there are considerable social problems in these communities and a failure to make use of health care. In contrast there was no difference in mortality between Canadian Africans and Chinese compared with white Canadians in Toronto.

Similarly in the UK, in both Birmingham and London, ethnic minorities (predominantly of African and Indian subcontinent decent) have not shown an increased risk of death, despite an increased risk of renal disease, compared with patients of white European descent. This probably reflects health benefits from universal access to education and medical care including free prescriptions for those on benefits, although poor compliance/adherence remains a significant risk factor for renal failure. These patients were managed in centres with considerable experience in managing lupus and studies have shown that outcomes, particularly of hospitalizations, are significantly improved in specialist centres including a reduced risk of death.

Causes of death

Factors influencing the increased risk of premature death in lupus patients are summarized in Table 3.7. It needs to be recognized that under-reporting of deaths associated with lupus as a direct or indirect cause is common. Several studies have shown that at most 50–60% of death certificates for lupus patients mention lupus as an underlying diagnosis. Poor ascertainment of deaths due to lupus in ethnic minorities has been shown to be more common than in white populations. From the data that does exist, it is clear that patients from the ethnic minorities have the highest risk of severe lupus, particularly renal disease, and the highest risk of dying from active lupus and end-stage renal disease. Renal disease is a recognized cause of increased death even in the non-lupus African American, Hispanic and Chinese populations. Comorbidities such as hypertension, diabetes, and obesity are common in the ethnic minorities and poor control of these conditions frequently contributes to deaths.

Table 3.7 Main risk factors influencing risk of premature death in lupus patients

Non-SLE factors	SLE factors	Treatment factors	Co-morbidities
Race/ethnicity	Age at diagnosis	Steroids	Hypertension
Sex	Time to diagnosis	Cyclophosphamide	Diabetes
Year of birth	Year of diagnosis	Hydroxychloroquine (protective)	Hypercholesterolaemia
Education	Renal involvement	Immunization	Obesity
Income	Severe disease activity	Adherence	Pre-existing atherosclerosis
Access to health care	Chronic damage		
Smoking			
Diet			
Housing			
Environment (climate, UV light, chemical exposure)			
Social support			
Public health			

Urowitz was the first to report in 1976 a bimodal pattern of death in lupus patients with deaths early in the disease course (≤5 years from diagnosis) mostly due to active lupus and infection. Deaths later in the disease course (5 years after diagnosis) were mostly due to cardiovascular disease and end-organ failure, though infection remained a significant cause of death.

In the SLICC mortality study published in 2006, there were 3.8 deaths per 1000 person-years of follow-up due to lupus and 4.1 deaths per 1000 person-years due to circulatory diseases which included all types of heart disease, arterial disease, and cerebrovascular accidents. For deaths due to these circulatory diseases, the SMR was 1.7 (95% CI, 1.5–1.9). For infections excluding pneumonias, the SMR was 5.0 (95% CI, 3.7–6.7) and for pneumonia specifically, the SMR was 2.6 (95% CI, 1.6–4.1). This highlights the significant role of infection in causing death in lupus patients. Renal disease which was mostly due to lupus was associated with the highest SMR in this cohort at 7.9 (95% CI, 5.5–11.0). The time when there was the highest risk of death was in first year after diagnosis with an SMR of 5.4 (4.7–6.3) and this probably reflects the dual problem of poorly controlled, active disease and the highest doses of steroids contributing to deaths from active disease and infection. The SMR was 2.8 (95% CI, 1.2–5.6) for non-Hodgkin's lymphoma, and for lung cancer it was 2.3 (95% CI, 1.6–3.0), but for cancer overall the SMR was 0.8 (95% CI, 0.6–1.0). More recent studies have highlighted that non-Hodgkin's lymphoma and lung cancer (especially in smokers) are increased in lupus patients (see Chapter 9, Management of special situations in SLE) but are still rare in absolute terms. There is no evidence that other cancers are a significant cause of death in lupus patients and this has been confirmed in the meta-analysis by Yurkovitch in 2014.

The Euro-Lupus project reported in 2009 that about 25% of deaths in lupus patients were due to active lupus, but there was a reduction in numbers between 1995 and 2000 (22%) compared with 1990 to 1995 (29%), and infections accounted for 29% and 17% of deaths in the same time period. They reported thromboses as the other main cause of death, occurring in 26%, with no change in the proportion over time and very few deaths due to malignancy (<7%). Other studies have not specifically reported deaths associated with thrombosis so it is difficult to compare this data with other studies.

In the recent UK study from Birmingham, published in 2014, with multi-ethnic patient data from 1989 to 2010, there were 37 deaths in 382 patients (92% female, 68% white) and an overall SMR of 2.0 (95% CI, 1.5–2.8). Despite widespread access to health care and education, the mean age (SD) at death was only 53.7 years (SD 17.4), over 25 years less than the mean age of death for the population of England and Wales. The mean disease duration at death was 6.9 years (SD 4.4). Infection was the commonest cause of death and accounted for 38% of deaths. Cardiovascular causes of death were found in 27.0%, malignancy in 14%, acute respiratory distress syndrome in 5%, active SLE in 5%, and about 3% of deaths were each due to pulmonary hypertension, cardiac tamponade, gastrointestinal bleed and alcoholic liver cirrhosis. As in the previous UK study from University College Hospital London, the risk of death was increased in those with significantly active lupus disease (high British Isles Lupus Assessment Group (BILAG) disease activity scores) that developed damage, particularly those with renal involvement, as had been found in other studies with different measures of disease activity. Treatment with cyclophosphamide also contributed to an increased risk of damage in these studies and has been shown to predispose to serious infection (Lertchaisataporn, 2013).

Neuro-psychiatric disease was also a predictor of damage in the Birmingham cohort and in the past was considered a risk factor for mortality in lupus patients. This has not been reported in many studies in the last two decades but a recent study from the Netherlands found that patients that have suffered from neuro-psychiatric lupus (NP-lupus) have a high risk of dying. They followed 169 patients with NP-lupus since 1989 and found the SMR was 9.5 (95% CI, 6.7–13.5). The most common causes of death in these patients was infection and NP-lupus, and anti-platelet therapy was protective with a hazard ratio of 0.22 (95% CI, 0.07–0.74). Diagnosis of acute confusional state and older age at diagnosis of NP-lupus were associated with increased hazard ratios in the multivariate analysis (3.38 and 1.06, respectively).

In other North European studies, such as the study by Voss published in 2013 covering the outcome of 215 predominantly white patients with lupus between 1995 and 2010 in Funen county, Denmark, cardiovascular disease was the commonest cause of death. This was first reported from Sweden by Bjornadal in 2004 with data from a much larger Swedish study with nearly 5000 patients, undertaken between 1964 and 1995. The overall SMR was 2.2 in the Danish study, with the highest SMR of 21.1 for those aged 20–29 in this population-based study that avoided the bias due to inclusion of only more severe cases seen in hospitals that occurs in some studies. The median age at death was 64 years. Cumulative survival rates were 93.6% at 5 years, 86.5% at 10 years, and 73% at 15 years. Cardiovascular events accounted for 32% of deaths, 16% were due to respiratory system disease, with 13% dying from malignancies. There were few deaths due to active lupus or infection except in the newly diagnosed. Renal disease was more common among the group of patients that died during the study period (50%), compared with those still alive at the end of the study (31%; $p = 0.034$). Thromboembolic events were also more common in the group of patients that died (50% vs 27%; $p = 0.008$). Hydroxychloroquine appeared to be protective as it was prescribed to 74% survivors, compared with 53% of deceased patients ($p = 0.015$).

In the Swedish study reported by Bjornadal in 2004, the SMR was 3.63 (95% CI, 3.49–3.78). All-cause mortality decreased from 1975 to 1995 due to a reduction in deaths attributed to SLE, but cardiovascular disease remained a major cause of death even in young patients in the last decade studied. Patients aged 20–39 at first discharge showed a reduction in mortality, with SMR 33.6 (95% CI, 24.3–45.3) before 1975 compared with SMR 14.2 (95% CI, 8.7–22.0) after 1984, but the SMR for deaths from coronary heart disease was 16.0 and showed no improvement over time.

A more recent study from Sweden published by Gustafsson in 2012 reported an even higher rate of cardiovascular deaths in a smaller cohort of 208 lupus patients (94% European Caucasians) recruited between 1995 and 1999 and followed up for 12 years. The mean age of death was 62 years in the 42 patients that died. The overall SMR was 2.4 (95% CI, 1.7–3.0) and 48% of deaths were due to cardiovascular disease. They found that traditional risk factors, apart from smoking, did not predict risk of cardiovascular mortality and found that inflammatory, endothelial, and thrombotic (anti-phospholipid) markers discriminated between those with favourable versus poor cardiovascular outcomes better.

Deaths due to cardiovascular and other circulatory disorders have not reduced in frequency over the last 20 years in European and other international studies and highlight the need to reduce risk factors for atherosclerosis including hypertension, hypercholesterolaemia, metabolic syndrome, medications such as steroids, and disease-related factors. Even when lupus is not the cause of death in European studies, an increased risk of death is observed in patients with increased damage, which occurs in those patients with a history of high disease activity especially in renal, neuropsychiatric, cardiopulmonary, and musculoskeletal systems.

The meta-analysis by Yurkovitch confirmed a roughly 3-fold increased risk of dying from cardiovascular disease, a 5-fold increased risk of dying from infection, and no significant increased risk of dying from malignancy in lupus patients. The risk of dying from renal disease was reported as being nearly 8-fold higher than expected. This was based on only one study that met the inclusion criteria for the meta-analysis and this was the SLICC mortality study discussed earlier in this section (Causes of death).

Further recent evidence for the impact of renal disease on mortality has come from a US study published by Sule in 2012 showing that patients with end-stage renal disease (ESRD) due to lupus were hospitalized more frequently and had a higher risk of death than adults with ESRD due to other causes (hazard ratio 1.89; 95% CI, 1.66–2.50). Children with lupus and ESRD also had higher rates of admission and mortality compared with children with ESRD due to other causes or adults with lupus and ESRD (hazard ratio 2.05; 95% CI, 1.79–2.34). Yap reported in 2012 that in 230 Chinese patients with lupus nephritis the 5-, 10-, and 20-year survival rates were 98.6%, 98.2%, and 90.5%. The cause of death was infection in 50% of patients, cardiovascular disease in 20.8%, and malignancy in 12.5%. The SMR in patients with renal involvement was 5.9; for those with ESRD it was 26.1; with malignancy, 12.9; and with cardiovascular disease, 13.6. These outcomes are better than those from a study in Hong Kong published by Mok in 2013, reporting that in 694 lupus patients followed from 1995 to 2011, the SMR was 4.8 for those without renal involvement (47%) and 9.0 for those with lupus nephritis (53%). The SMR was 9.8 for proliferative lupus nephritis and 6.1 for membranous lupus nephritis. End-stage renal disease developed in 24 patients and they had an SMR of 63.1. In a study from Barbados published by Flower in 2012, the 5-year survival was only 68% in patients with nephritis compared with 80% overall for the 183 new cases of lupus recruited between 2000 and 2009 (47% with nephritis at presentation).

Conclusions

Lupus is a disease that is more common than is generally recognized even in white populations. It occurs most frequently in women but may be missed in men who are less likely to report milder symptoms and tend to present with more severe disease. There is a significantly higher risk of developing the disease in people of African, Hispanic, and Asian (especially Chinese) descent and recent studies have highlighted an increased incidence and prevalence in First Nation Canadians, American Indians, Alaska Natives, and Australian Aborigines. All of these ethnic minorities appear to develop lupus with a more severe phenotype, often with renal involvement and at an earlier age than white people of North European descent.

Although deaths due to lupus now seem to be less common than 50–60 years ago, particularly in North American and European countries, deaths due to renal lupus remain a significant problem in the ethnic minorities especially those of African, Hispanic and Chinese descent around the world, and the outcome is worst in poor patients with sub-optimal medical care. Infection is a universal, common but potentially preventable and treatable cause of death. Cardiovascular disease remains a significant cause of premature death in European and North American patients that should also be preventable.

Management needs to be targeted at reducing factors that increase the risk of lupus disease activity, damage, and mortality. This requires raising awareness about the disease, as early diagnosis and the swift institution of appropriate therapy to reduce disease activity will reduce the development of chronic damage and the associated risk of subsequent premature death. Although there is data emphasizing the importance of early renal biopsy to ensure optimal therapy for lupus nephritis with immunosuppressants, as this improves the chances of complete response and significantly reduces the risk of late end-stage renal disease, there are still patients with proteinuria that are monitored without definitive treatment for far longer than is ideal.

Many women come into contact with health professionals while preparing for and during pregnancy and it is important to ensure that proteinuria is screened for in these individuals and that resolution after pregnancy is confirmed or investigated. Cyclophosphamide should be avoided now that there are safer immunosuppressive drugs with less risk of infertility, malignancy, and infection. Hydroxychloroquine and anti-platelet therapy may provide protection against death in lupus patients. Corticosteroids are important in reducing disease activity quickly, but need to be used with caution in view of their many known adverse effects that increase the accumulation of damage, particularly cardiovascular disease, and the risk of death. These issues are discussed further in Chapter 6 (Conventional treatments in SLE).

Further reading

Abu-Shakra M, Urowitz MB, Gladman DD, Gough J. Mortality studies in systemic lupus erythematosus. Results from a single center. I. Causes of death. *J Rheumatol* 1995;22:1259–64.

Bernatsky S, Boivin JF, Joseph L, et al. Mortality in systemic lupus erythematosus. *Arthritis Rheum* 2006;54(8):2550–7.

Bjornadal L, Yin L, Granath F, Klareskog L, Ekbom A. Cardiovascular disease a hazard despite improved prognosis in patients with systemic lupus erythematosus: results from a Swedish population based study 1964–1995. *J Rheumatol* 2004;31:713–9.

Cervera R, Khamashta MA, Hughes GR. The Euro-lupus project: epidemiology of systemic lupus erythematosus in Europe. *Lupus* 2009;18:869–74.

Fernandez M, Alarcon GS, Calvo-Alen J, et al. A multiethnic, multicenter cohort of patients with systemic lupus erythematosus (SLE) as a model for the study of ethnic disparities in SLE. *Arthritis Rheum* 2007;57:576–84.

Flower C, Hennis AJ, Hambleton IR, Nicholson GD, Liang MH. Systemic lupus erythematosus in an African Caribbean population: incidence, clinical manifestations, and survival in the Barbados National Lupus Registry. *Arthritis Care Res* (Hoboken) 2012;64:1151–8.

Gonzalez LA, Toloza SM, Alarcon GS. Impact of race and ethnicity in the course and outcome of systemic lupus erythematosus. Rheum Dis Clin North Am 2014 August;40(3):433–454.

Gustafsson JT, Simard JF, Gunnarsson I, et al. Risk factors for cardiovascular mortality in patients with systemic lupus erythematosus, a prospective cohort study. *Arthritis Res Ther* 2012;14:R46.

Johnson AE, Gordon C; Palmer RG, Bacon PA. The prevalence and incidence of systemic lupus erythematosus in Birmingham, England. Relationship to ethnicity and country of birth. *Arthritis Rheum* 1995;38:551–8.

Lim SS, Bayakly AR, Helmick CG, Gordon C, Easley KA, Drenkard C. The incidence and prevalence of systemic lupus erythematosus, 2002–2004: The Georgia Lupus Registry. *Arthritis Rheumatol* 2014;66:357–68.

Lim SS, Drenkard C, McCune WJ, et al. Population-based lupus registries: advancing our epidemiologic understanding. *Arthritis Rheum* 2009;61:1462–6.

Rees F, Doherty M, Grainge M, Davenport G, Lanyon P, Zhang W. The incidence and prevalence of systemic lupus erythematosus in the UK, 1999–2012. *Ann Rheum Dis* 2014 September 29. doi: 10.1136/annrheumdis-2014-206334 (Epub ahead of print).

Somers EC, Marder W, Cagnoli P, et al. Population-based incidence and prevalence of systemic lupus erythematosus: the Michigan lupus epidemiology and surveillance program. *Arthritis Rheumatol* 2014;66:369–78.

Urowitz MB, Gladman DD, Tom BD, Ibanez D, Farewell VT. Changing patterns in mortality and disease outcomes for patients with systemic lupus erythematosus. *J Rheumatol* 2008;35:2152–8.

Watson L, Leone V, Pilkington C. Disease activity, severity, and damage in the UK Juvenile-Onset Systemic Lupus Erythematosus Cohort. *Arthritis Rheum* 2012;64:2356–65.

Yee CS, Su L, Toescu V, et al. Birmingham SLE cohort: outcomes of a large inception cohort followed for up to 21 years. *Rheumatology* (Oxford) 2015;54:836–43.

Chapter 4

Clinical features of systemic lupus erythematosus

Ben Rhodes and Caroline Gordon

Key points

- SLE most commonly presents with inflammatory arthritis, rashes, and lymphopenia, although involvement of any organ system is possible.
- Fatigue, arthralgia, and myalgia are common, but they are non-specific symptoms and should not be considered diagnostic features.
- Infection is an important differential diagnosis, particularly in patients with fever and lymphadenopathy: it should always be excluded by rigorous clinical evaluation.
- Lupus nephritis is often asymptomatic and regular screening by urinary protein quantification is important to ensure early detection and treatment of this disease manifestation.
- The assessment of neurological symptoms and signs can be challenging and requires careful evaluation including detailed investigation before attribution to lupus can be made, with consideration of thrombotic as well as inflammatory aetiology.

Introduction

A notable feature of systemic lupus erythematosus (SLE or lupus) is its variability: in the clinical presentation, in the involvement of different organ systems and in the pattern of disease activity. While many of the individual features of lupus can occur as single organ diseases (including cutaneous, renal, and haematological manifestations), by its very definition lupus is characterized by a number of different autoimmune features affecting different systems. These features can occur in any combination, either synchronously or sequentially, so that patients carrying the diagnostic label of SLE can differ almost entirely in clinical characteristics. Patterns of disease activity can also vary, with some patients maintaining chronic disease activity despite treatment, others experiencing recurrent disease flares with intervening periods of low disease activity, and some entering prolonged remission after a relatively short initial period of activity.

Musculoskeletal and mucocutaneous disease manifestations are the most common, but it is involvement of the kidneys and the central nervous and cardiorespiratory systems, along with an increased risk of infection, that accounts for most mortality and morbidity. In addition to clinical features that are clearly immune-mediated and related to disease activity, lupus is also associated with features that, while impacting greatly on the patient, are relatively non-specific: fatigue is foremost in this group of symptoms. A good grasp of the clinical features felt to be attributable to active lupus can be achieved by reviewing the multisystem scoring system used in the British Isles Lupus Assessment Group (BILAG) disease activity index. We have deliberately structured this chapter to consider clinical features and their differential diagnosis when relevant within their BILAG domain. We have focussed discussion on the clinical features of primary active SLE rather than features due to disease damage, complications, and therapy.

Constitutional features

Commonly observed constitutional features in lupus include fever, fatigue, weight loss, and lymphadenopathy. Fatigue is a subjective sensation, previously described as, 'an uncommon, abnormal, or extreme whole body tiredness, disproportionate to, or unrelated to, activity or exertion'. This subjectiveness, combined with inconsistent definitions applied across studies and different instruments to measure fatigue, make the literature difficult to interpret. It is nonetheless clear that fatigue is common; with studies suggesting 53–80% of patients with SLE have fatigue as one of their key symptoms. This appears similar to the prevalence of fatigue seen in patients with other chronic inflammatory diseases such as multiple sclerosis and rheumatoid arthritis. However, it should be borne in mind that population studies also suggest a high prevalence of fatigue in the general population with prevalent fatigue of approximately 40%, and 20% reporting long-lasting fatigue.

It has been reported that 40–60% of patients with lupus develop a fever during the course of their illness and it is a common cause of hospitalization. While it can be seen as a feature of active lupus it is extremely important to consider the differential diagnosis; in particular infection. Infection may be more severe in patients with lupus due to a number of factors including the immunological consequences of active disease (such as hypocomplementaemia) or its treatment with steroids and other immune suppressants. Infection is a leading cause of mortality in lupus, accounting for a quarter of all deaths. Infections may include typical respiratory and urinary infection, tuberculosis, or opportunistic infections such as *Pneumocystis jirovecii*. To complicate the evaluation it should also be considered that infections themselves appear to be associated with the onset of lupus or disease exacerbations. A recent study proposed that an algorithm incorporating fever duration, serum C-reactive protein, and anti-dsDNA antibody levels performed reasonably well as a discriminator of infection (higher CRP/shorter temperature duration and lower anti-dsDNA levels) over active lupus, but this is no substitute for detailed clinical evaluation by an experienced physician.

Lymphadenopathy, usually fluctuant, occurring early in the course of the disease and in association with other disease features, is recognized in lupus. As with fever, infection is an important differential diagnosis. Kikuchi–Fujimoto disease (necrotizing lymphadenitis) is another condition that presents with tender lymphadenopathy and often profound constitutional symptoms. About a third of patients with this condition go on to develop typical lupus. Lymphoma and solid organ malignancy should also be considered in the patient presenting with progressive lymphadenopathy. Lymphoma is more common in lupus and if in doubt a biopsy and histological evaluation should be undertaken (see Chapter 9, Management of special situations).

Weight loss can certainly occur in patients with active lupus and is a 'scorable' item in the BILAG and the systemic lupus activity measure-revised (SLAM-R) disease activity indices. It often occurs along with other constitutional features discussed in this section and the same requirement to exclude infection and malignancy applies to weight loss.

Musculoskeletal disease

Involvement of the musculoskeletal system is undoubtedly one of the commonest features of active lupus and affects over 80% of patients. Disease involving the joints, peri-articular structures and muscle has been described. Arthralgia, by which we mean joint pain that is not accompanied by objective clinical evidence of inflammation, but is associated with significant early morning stiffness consistent with an underlying inflammatory process, is the most common musculoskeletal manifestation. Ultrasound evaluation may reveal sub-clinical joint inflammation in some of these patients. Frank arthritis presents as transient or persistent symmetrical joint inflammation, with the small joints of the hands (Figure 4.1 (see colour version on inside cover)) and the knees most commonly affected. A typical picture of early morning stiffness, joint erythema, reduced range of movement, tenderness and swelling is often seen, but the swelling is usually not as prominent as in rheumatoid arthritis. Some patients will have arthralgia associated with osteoarthritis that is more prominent on activity and should not be confused with lupus arthritis.

Tenosynovial inflammation is also common in lupus and again has been confirmed in ultrasound studies. Tendon rupture, including Achilles, patellar, and hand tendons, is rare but well described, with long-term steroid use also contributing to this risk.

Jaccoud's arthropathy affects about 5% of patients with lupus, and is characterized by hand deformities including limited extension with ulnar deviation of the metacarpophalangeal joints, swan-neck and boutonniere' deformities, and Z-shaped thumbs (Figure 4.2 (see colour version on inside cover)). Classically Jaccoud's deformities are reducible and, in general, radiographic bony erosions are not seen. It is generally thought that Jaccoud's arthropathy is a consequence of low-grade synovial and tenosynovial inflammation leading

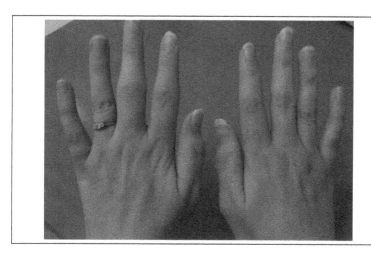

Figure 4.1 Inflammatory polyarthritis of the hands affecting the proximal interphalangeal and metacarpophalangeal joints in a patient with lupus. (See colour version on inside cover.)

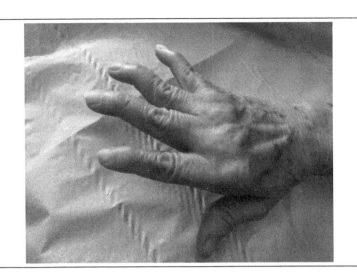

Figure 4.2 Jaccoud's arthropathy with reducible swan-neck deformities affecting the hand and involvement of the thumb in a lupus patient. (See colour version on inside cover.)

to laxity of the joint capsule and tendons, with the subsequently imbalanced muscular contraction leading to deformity. It should be noted that this can recur after joint surgery.

A small number of lupus patients (perhaps <5%) develop a deforming arthropathy, with radiological erosions that are indistinguishable from those seen in rheumatoid arthritis. The use of ultrasound or MRI increases the detection of these erosions to over 10%. Most, but not all, studies show an association of erosive disease with the presence of anti-cyclic citrullinated peptide (anti-CCP) antibodies. Whether this is a true subset of lupus, or whether it is a co-occurrence of lupus and rheumatoid arthritis is uncertain—the term 'rhupus' has been applied to this group of patients.

Myalgias and muscle biopsy abnormalities appear quite common in patients with lupus (typically a lymphocytic vasculitis with Type II muscle fibre atrophy); but true myositis is unusual (<5%), to the extent that it is generally considered to be a lupus/myositis 'overlap' syndrome usually associated with anti-ribonucleoprotein (anti-RNP) antibodies, rather than a specific manifestation of lupus itself. Fibromyalgia may occur in up to 15% of lupus patients but must not be confused with lupus disease activity.

Avascular necrosis is best considered an item of lupus damage rather than a feature of active disease. It is a recognized complication that affects 4–15% of patients. It presents with progressive mechanical joint pain most commonly of the hip (Figure 4.3), but can affect the shoulder, knee, wrist, and ankle, and may be unilateral or bilateral. Steroids may contribute to this risk, but this condition remains poorly understood with non-steroid factors at play including the disease activity for which steroids are used and possibly thrombosis.

Mucocutaneous disease

A wide range of cutaneous lesions are seen in systemic lupus erythematosus. The most recent classification scheme (the Düsseldorf classification, see Box 4.1) divides these

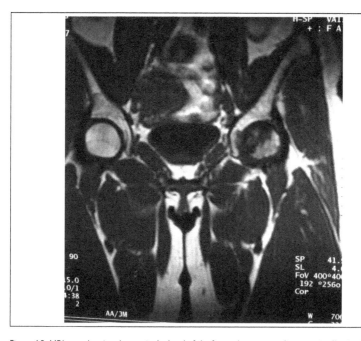

Figure 4.3 MRI scan showing changes in the head of the femur due to avascular necrosis affecting the left hip with minimal change in the right hip.

into lupus-specific lesions and lesions that are also seen in other diseases. Lupus-specific lesions are then subdivided into acute, subacute, and chronic forms, with the placement of the rare lupus tumidus as an intermittent lupus erythematosus subtype remaining an area of some uncertainty. The recent Systemic Lupus International Collaborating Clinics (SLICC) Classification Criteria for SLE include all the lupus-specific rashes. The older American College of Rheumatology criteria only includes three cutaneous features: malar rash, discoid rash, and photosensitivity; meaning that some clear-cut lupus rashes get excluded and the rather non-specific photosensitivity contributes, even though it is often associated with a malar or discoid rash already recorded. While many patients with lupus undoubtedly have photosensitivity, photosensitivity also occurs in other diseases, for example polymorphic light eruption.

Skin lesions are very common in lupus, both at presentation and throughout the course of the illness. Isolated skin disease (cutaneous lupus erythematosus) is more common than systemic lupus but is considered as a separate entity, albeit with similar treatment options.

Acute cutaneous lupus (ACLE) includes the iconic malar or 'butterfly' rash (Figure 4.4a (see colour version on inside cover)), and also a more widespread maculopapular rash. The typical malar rash consists of symmetrical macules, often becoming confluent across the bridge of the nose and sparing the nasolabial folds. The rash can be oedematous and slightly raised, or covered in a fine scale and it is important clinically to distinguish it from the common facial rashes of rosacea and seborrhoeic dermatitis. The rash generally lasts from hours to weeks and can precede other features of active

Box 4.1 The 'Dusseldorf' 2003 classification of cutaneous lupus

Lupus erythematosus specific skin lesions:
- Acute cutaneous lupus erythematosus (ACLE)
  a) Localized ACLE—typically a 'butterfly' malar rash
  b) Generalized ACLE
  c) Bullous lupus/toxic epidermal necrolysis-like.
- Subacute cutaneous lupus erythematosus (SCLE)
  a) Annular variant
  b) Papulosquamous variant.
- Chronic cutaneous lupus erythematosus (CCLE)
  a) Discoid lupus
  b) Lupus profundus
  c) Chilblain lupus.

Lupus erythematosus non-specific skin lesions include:
- Leucocytoclastic vasculitis
- Livido reticularis
- Periungual telangiectasia
- Raynaud's phenomenon
- Non-scarring alopecia
- Calcinosis and scleroderma-like changes
- Non-specific bullous lesions.

Kuhn A, Ruzicka T. Classification of cutaneous lupus erythematosus. In: Kuhn A, Lehmann P, Ruzicka T. eds. Cutaneous lupus erythematosus. Berlin: Springer Verlag; 2004:53–58.

lupus or be present during active systemic disease. Generalized, maculopapular acute cutaneous lupus is less common but is similarly associated with active disease. It is symmetrical and often itchy. It is generally widespread but can be worse on sun-exposed areas. On the hands it can affect the palms and periungual area but, in contrast to dermatomyositis, spares the skin overlying the dorsum of the small joints.

Mucocutaneous lesions in lupus are common and considered part of the ACLE spectrum. Painful ulcers are particularly seen on the lips, buccal mucosa and palate, although

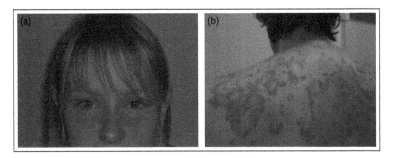

Figure 4.4 a) Classical photosensitive butterfly or malar rash on the face due to lupus. b) Subacute cutaneous lupus rash on the back showing annular lesions that consist of scaly, coalescing, erythematous plaques with central clearing.

they may occur elsewhere in the mouth and in the nostrils. Rarely, acute cutaneous lupus can develop into severe bullous or toxic-epidermal necrolysis-like forms. ACLE resolves without scarring, although post-inflammatory pigmentation or depigmentation can occur, which is particularly noticeable with darker skin.

Subacute cutaneous lupus (SCLE) has two variants. Slightly more common is an annular variant which consists of scaly, coalescing, annular erythematous plaques with central clearing (Figure 4.4b (see colour version on inside cover)). The papulosquamous variant consists of erythematous, slightly scaly lesions that can resemble psoriasis, or eczema, or pityriasis. SCLE generally occurs on the upper body but sparing the face and scalp, and like ACLE has a predilection for sun-exposed areas. It also resolves without scarring, but with a risk of post-inflammatory pigmentation or depigmentation. There is a strong association between SCLE and the presence of anti-Ro and anti-La antibodies, and patients with this rash often have a generally milder systemic disease course.

Chronic cutaneous lupus also includes a number of distinct variants of which discoid lupus erythematosus is by far the most common. The lesions of discoid lupus consist of well-demarcated, erythematous scaly macules that enlarge into indurated plaques with adherent scale that can mimic psoriasis. Chronic lesions become atrophic and scarred. Typically the ears and scalp are affected and, when plaques involve the hair follicles a patchy alopecia (Figure 4.5) develops. The arms and hands can also be involved and rarely, the mucosal surfaces. Discoid lupus tends to occur in older patients than ACLE and SCLE, and only about 10% of patients with discoid lupus erythematosus actually develop systemic lupus at all. Rarer forms of chronic cutaneous lupus include: lupus profundus, which is a panniculitis causing deep, painful indurated nodules; and chilblain lupus which causes cool, painful, purple nodules in cold-exposed extremities.

Other mucocutaneous features of lupus include oral and nasal ulcers and Raynaud's phenomenon, a reflex vasoconstriction affecting the extremities. Diffuse alopecia is more common than the patchy alopecia associated with a discoid rash, and is usually reversible with treatment. It is important to exclude hypothyroidism in patients with diffuse alopecia.

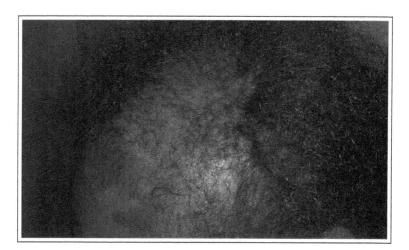

Figure 4.5 Patchy alopecia with scarring of the scalp due to discoid lupus.

The cutaneous lupus erythematosus disease area and severity index (CLASI) is a dedicated scoring system for cutaneous lupus that can be used in clinical practise or in research studies. It captures skin involvement due to active disease and chronic damage.

Renal disease

Approximately 25–55% of lupus patients will get renal disease (lupus nephritis). Just like lupus as a whole, the prevalence varies significantly with race and ethnicity, being much more prevalent in patients of Chinese, South Asian, and African-American/Caribbean ancestries than in those of Northern European ancestry. Lupus nephritis is twice as prevalent in children presenting with lupus as compared with adults. It is associated with more severe disease and reduced survival compared with non-nephritis lupus. The recent SLICC classification criteria recognize that lupus nephritis, in an appropriate immunological context, may occur in isolation and is consistent with a classification (and clinical diagnosis) of SLE.

The classification of lupus nephritis is generally made on histological appearance, with the most recent scheme being the International Society of Nephrology/Renal Pathology Society (ISN/RPS) 2003 classification (Table 4.1 and Chapter 5, Figure 5.4 and colour version on inside cover). This scheme recognizes that lupus nephritis is

Table 4.1 International Society of Nephrology/Renal Pathology Society (ISN/RPS) 2003 classification of lupus nephritis

Class I	**Minimal mesangial proliferative lupus nephritis**
	Normal glomeruli by light microscopy, but mesangial immune deposits by immunofluorescence
Class II	**Mesangial proliferative lupus nephritis**
	Purely mesangial hypercellularity or matrix expansion by light microscopy, with mesangial immune deposits. No subepithelial or subendothelial deposits by light microscopy.
Class III	**Focal lupus nephritis**
	Active or inactive, segmental or global endo- or extracapillary glomerulonephritis involving <50% of all glomeruli, typically with focal subendothelial immune deposits. Mesangial alterations may or may not be present.
Class IV	**Diffuse lupus nephritis**
	Active or inactive, segmental or global endo- or extracapillary glomerulonephritis involving >50% or all glomeruli, typically with focal subendothelial immune deposits. Mesangial alterations may or may not be present.
	Divided into IV-S when >50% of glomeruli have segmental lesions (involving less than half the glomerular tuft) and IV-G when >50% of glomeruli have global lesions.
Class V	**Membranous lupus nephritis**
	Global or segmental subepithelial immune deposits, with or without mesangial alteration.
	May occur in conjunction with class II or IV in which case both are diagnosed.
Class VI	**Advanced sclerosis**
	>90% glomeruli globally sclerosed with no residual activity.

Weening JJ, D'Agati VD, Schwartz MM et al. The classification of glomerulonephritis in systemic lupus erythematosus revisited. JASN 2004;15:241–250.

primarily a disease of the renal glomerulus, which is caused by immune complex deposition and subsequent inflammation leading to glomerular dysfunction.

Most lupus nephritis is initially asymptomatic, with normal renal function and is therefore detected on the basis of urinary abnormalities. The most common abnormality is a rise in urinary protein. Proteinuria greater than 0.5 g/24 hours or a protein:creatinine or albumin:creatinine ratio greater than 50 mg/mmol is considered 'significant' for classification purposes. Nephritis may also be associated with an 'active urinary sediment', consisting of red and white blood cells in the urine and cellular casts (with no bacteriuria). The isolated presence of low levels of urinary white cells ('sterile pyuria') is a common finding in patients with lupus and, in the context of normal urine protein, otherwise inactive sediment, and inactive systemic disease, should not be attributed to lupus as this is usually associated with urinary or vaginal infection which is not necessarily symptomatic.

The key classes of nephritis seen on biopsy (see Chapter 5, Laboratory tests and investigations, Figure 5.4 and colour version on inside cover) are generally, but not exclusively, associated with a clinical picture which reflects the nature of glomerular dysfunction which, in turn, depends largely on the location of immune complex deposition. Class V nephritis is typically associated with heavy proteinuria (sometimes >5 g/24 hours) and patients may develop the clinical features of nephrotic syndrome which include marked peripheral oedema, hypertension, hypercoagulability, and hypercholesterolaemia. Class III and particularly Class IV nephritis typically present with lower levels of proteinuria, but are associated with an active urinary sediment and have a greater propensity to deteriorating renal function, that in rare cases is rapid. Class I and II nephritis is usually associated only with mild or modest proteinuria, that has minimal prognostic significance. Advanced disease (Class VI) is typically associated with severe scarring and chronic/end-stage kidney disease with varying levels of proteinuria.

The exact prevalence of chronic kidney disease (CKD—a permanent impairment of renal function) in patients with lupus nephritis is difficult to estimate. The presence of CKD and its progression to end-stage renal disease (ESRD—renal failure requiring renal replacement therapy) is particularly seen in patients who are non-compliant with medication, present late, fail to achieve remission, or have frequently relapsing disease. The prevalence of ESRD is considerably higher in high risk populations of African ancestry. It has recently been documented that the incidence of ESRD attributable to lupus in the US has tripled over the last 30 years.

The development of CKD and ESRD is closely linked to a failure to induce effective disease remission. Outcomes appear to be best in patients in whom definitive immunosuppression is initiated early, usually preceded by renal biopsy to provide both diagnostic certainty and a measure of renal activity and damage. Since early detection and treatment is critical to optimizing the chances of achieving this, a key task of the lupus physician is to ensure effective urine monitoring is in place for all lupus patients (as a minimum: six monthly for stable patients with no history of nephritis, and three monthly for those with a history of nephritis).

Haematological disease

Haematological disease, including anaemia, immune-mediated thrombocytopenia, leucopenia, and clotting abnormalities due to anti-phospholipid antibodies are all common in lupus. The differential diagnosis of cytopenias in discussed further in Chapter 5 (Laboratory tests and investigations) but includes immune-mediated destruction, medication effects, and non-specific effects of chronic inflammatory disease. Distinguishing active disease from drug side-effects can be a challenging, but important, aspect of management. Anaemia in lupus is most commonly due to bone marrow suppression by chronic inflammatory disease, often exacerbated by underlying iron deficiency, and contributes to the fatigue experienced by lupus patients. Much less common, but potentially more serious is autoimmune haemolytic anaemia due to antibody-mediated peripheral destruction of red cells. Haemoglobin usually drops quickly and patients have a positive direct Coombs' test. Pure red cell aplasia, whilst rare, can also occur, presumably when antibodies target early lineage bone marrow cells.

A mild, asymptomatic, reduction in platelet count ($100-150 \times 10^9/mL$) is commonly seen in lupus, often, but not always, associated with the presence of antiphospholipid antibodies. A profound reduction in platelets, associated with bleeding (commonly cutaneous petechiae and bleeding of the gums), is much rarer and can predate the development of SLE so that the patient is initially treated for isolated immune thrombocytopenic purpura (ITP) before developing other features leading to a formal lupus diagnosis. Potentially even more serious is thrombotic thrombocytopenic purpura (TTP) in which low platelets and a coagulopathy occur in the presence of disseminated intravascular thrombosis with impaired renal function. This is a rare but potentially fatal complication that requires rapid diagnosis (blood film, platelet count, and markers of haemolysis) and treatment with high dose corticosteroids and plasma exchange.

Mild lymphopenia ($0.5-1.0 \times 10^9/mL$) is an extremely common and generally asymptomatic observation in lupus. A more significant reduction in lymphocytes or other cells of myeloid or lymphoid lineage is less common and rarely associated with infectious complication. Mild leucopenia may, in part, reflect migration of cells out of the vascular compartment as part of the abnormal immune response in lupus. More severe leucopenia is due to immune-mediated destruction.

Antiphospholipid syndrome is diagnosed in patients in whom a history of thrombosis, late pregnancy miscarriage, or recurrent early pregnancy miscarriage is associated with persistent antiphospholipid antibodies. These are either detected directly as anti-cardiolipin or anti-β2-glycoprotein-1 antibodies or their presence is inferred from a positive lupus anti-coagulant test. Antiphospholipid syndrome can occur as a primary autoimmune disease or in association with lupus. Thrombosis can affect the venous circulation and present, for example as a deep vein thrombosis, pulmonary embolus, renal vein thrombosis, or Budd–Chiari syndrome. Alternatively, it can affect the arterial circulation and present as a clinical obvious cerebral infarct or infarct in any other arterial territory. It may also present as a syndrome of cerebral small-vessel ischaemia due to recurrent small infarcts which in severe cases can cause significant cognitive dysfunction and memory loss. While, even in untreated patients, thromboses usually occur sporadically, some patients develop an aggressive thrombotic disorder in which multiple sites are involved simultaneously or over a short period of time. This is termed catastrophic antiphospholipid syndrome (CAPS).

Numerous non-thrombotic manifestations have also been associated with the presence of anti-phospholipid antibodies, including cardiac valve vegetations; demyelinating and other neurological syndromes including migraine; livedo reticularis; and leg ulceration. Proving causation is difficult because these conditions are also seen in patients with lupus without antiphospholipid antibodies or, in the case of migraine, commonly within the general population. In addition, antiphospholipid antibodies are also reasonably common (approximately 1%) in the general population in individuals with no history of disease, thrombotic or otherwise. This remains a hotly debated field.

Neuropsychiatric disease

The American College of Rheumatology (ACR) classification criteria for SLE only include psychosis and seizures, however, many other clinical features may develop in this system. The term neuropsychiatric lupus is used to describe a range of neurological and psychiatric syndromes that are observed in patients with SLE. The ACR developed a standard nomenclature (Table 4.2a) and case definitions that highlight the 12 central and seven peripheral features that are most commonly seen in lupus patients (although some are rare in practice).

The mechanisms underlying neuropsychiatric lupus are incompletely understood, but two broad neuropathological elements are likely to be important. Firstly a non-inflammatory vasculopathy, perhaps mediated in part by anti-phospholipid antibodies or immune complex deposition is likely to underlie the majority of focal neurological syndromes (such as stroke) and some diffuse syndromes (such as

Table 4.2 Neuropsychiatric syndromes in lupus (ACR definition and suggested modifications)

a) American College of Rheumatology defined syndromes[a]

Central nervous system	Peripheral nervous system
• Aseptic meningitis	• Guillain–Barré syndrome
• Cerebrovascular disease	• Autonomic disorder
• Demyelinating syndrome	• Mononeuropathy
• Headache	• Myasthenia gravis
• Movement disorder	• Cranial neuropathy
• Myelopathy	• Plexopathy
• Seizure disorder	• Polyneuropathy (EMG confirmation)
• Acute confusional state	
• Anxiety disorder	
• Cognitive dysfunction	
• Mood disorder	
• Psychosis	

b) Ainiala's modified criteria (objective disease only)[b]

• Aseptic meningitis	• Guillain Barré syndrome
• Cerebrovascular disease	• Autonomic disorder
• Demyelinating syndrome	• Mononeuropathy
• Movement disorder	• Myasthenia gravis
• Myelopathy	• Cranial neuropathy
• Seizure disorder	• Plexopathy
• Acute confusional state	• EMG confirmed polyneuropathy
• Moderate or severe cognitive dysfunction	
• Severe depression	
• Psychosis	

[a]The American College of Rheumatology nomenclature and case definitions for neuropsychiatric lupus syndromes. Arthritis Rheum 1999;42:599–608.

[b]The American College of Rheumatology nomenclature and case definitions for neuropsychiatric lupus syndromes. Arthritis Rheum 1999, 42:599–608, Wiley; Ainiala H, Hietaharju A, Loukkola J et al. Validity of the new American College of Rheumatology criteria for neuropsychiatric lupus syndromes: a population-based evaluation. Arthritis Rheum 2001 45:419–434, Wiley.

Abbreviations: EMG: electromyography.

cognitive dysfunction). Histologically, non-inflammatory vascular disease with associated micro-infarctions appears to be the commonest finding in neuropsychiatric lupus and true cerebral vasculitis is rare. Secondly, an immune-mediated inflammatory process with contribution from specific anti-neuronal antibodies, cytokines, increased blood–brain barrier permeability and intrathecal immune complex formation is likely to underlie the majority of diffuse neurological syndromes (such as psychosis and acute confusion).

Even if applying ACR standardized case definitions, estimates for the prevalence of neuropsychiatric lupus differ dramatically (from less than 40% to over 90%) and there are a number of possible reasons for this discrepancy. Firstly, none of the ACR neurological syndromes are unique to lupus and many, such as headache and depression, are quite common in the general population, leading to low specificity. By modifying the criteria to exclude milder and more subjective neurological features (Table 4.2b) the specificity for neuropsychiatric lupus increases considerably from 46% to 93%. Secondly, there is the issue of deciding whether a neuropsychiatric syndrome is directly attributable to active lupus, or is a coincidental co-occurrence, or is related to complications of disease or therapy. This question is important not only from a research perspective, but also as a key element of clinical decision-making that will impact on treatment choices. There is no test that can definitively determine whether a neuropsychiatric event is directly due to lupus. Factors which suggest attribution include general SLE disease activity, a past history of neuropsychiatric events, and the presence of anti-phospholipid antibodies. Efforts have been made to create and validate formal neuropsychiatric lupus attribution algorithms, but the specificity and sensitivity are insufficient to replace the careful judgement of an experienced clinician.

A detailed discussion of each neurological manifestation is beyond the scope of this chapter, but we would make some general observations.

Headache and depression

Although headache is commonly reported in lupus patients, and indeed 'lupus headache' is a specific item in the SLE disease activity index (SLEDAI) and the BILAG disease activity index, large studies suggest that headache is no more prevalent in lupus patients than the general population, nor is it associated with general disease activity. Most patients have 'normal' tension headaches or migraine. The concept of 'lupus headache' is in doubt and should never be recorded on the indices unless very severe and persistent. It is essential in the correct clinical context, to investigate for syndromes such as sub-arachnoid haemorrhage, aseptic meningitis or venous sinus thrombosis (see Chapter 5, Laboratory tests and investigations). Similarly depression is very common in the general population and there are no specific features to distinguish depression in lupus.

Psychosis

Acute psychosis due to lupus is rare (~2%) but presents with a similar spectrum of features to paranoid schizophrenia, including delusions and auditory hallucinations. It is important to exclude psychosis induced by high-dose corticosteroid therapy and 'recreational' psychoactive drugs.

Demyelination including transverse myelitis

This is rare, affecting <5% of patients, often in patients with positive antiphospholipid antibodies and can be indistinguishable from multiple sclerosis. It is generally agreed that lupus and multiple sclerosis very rarely co-exist and, in the absence of strong evidence for lupus, the latter diagnosis may be more likely, but MRI scan appearance may be helpful (see Chapter 5, Laboratory tests and investigations). Transverse myelitis can present with paraplegia or quadriplegia depending on the level and can recur at higher levels over time. Long-segment myelitis associated with optic neuropathy is typical of neuromyelitis optica (Devic's disease) and should trigger testing for aquaporin-4 antibodies.

Neuropathy

A mild sensorimotor peripheral neuropathy is the commonest peripheral neurological syndrome in lupus, often not clearly associated with active disease. Autonomic neuropathies, mononeuritis multiplex, and acute demyelinating polyneuropathies have all been described.

Cognitive dysfunction

Cognitive dysfunction is a concept which incorporates memory, learning, information processing, and expression. Subjective cognitive dysfunction ('brain fog') is a very commonly reported symptom in patients with lupus, but lacks reproducibility on objective testing. Unfortunately formal neuropsychological tests are time-consuming and require expert interpretation making them unusable or unavailable in routine practice for most physicians.

Differential diagnosis and the importance of investigations in patients with neuro-psychiatric manifestations

See also Chapter 5, Laboratory tests and investigations.

The European League Against Rheumatism (EULAR) recommendations for the management of neuropsychiatric lupus recommend that: 'the evaluation of SLE patients with (new) signs or symptoms suggestive of neuropsychiatric disease is comparable to that in non-SLE patients who present with the same manifestations'. For example, intracranial infection may need to be excluded through lumbar puncture and evaluation of cerebrospinal fluid for viral infection; confusion and psychosis may need a thorough drug history and evaluation of metabolic status; neuropathy may need evaluation of vitamin B_{12} status; seizures may require and electroencephalogram, and so on to identify or exclude all potential non-lupus causes.

Magnetic resonance imaging (MRI) with angiography (MRA) is usually performed to exclude structural lesions, cerebral ischaemia, and venous sinus thrombosis. The commonest finding is of multiple, small, fixed lesions in the subcortical and periventricular white matter. These are often attributed to small vessel disease but are not specific for lupus. Functional techniques such as positron emission tomography (PET) and single photon emission computerized tomography (SPECT) have been reported to show abnormalities in cerebral lupus, but their specificity and applicability to routine practice are still uncertain.

Cardiorespiratory disease

Lupus can affect all parts of the respiratory system including the pleura, respiratory muscles, lung parenchyma and vasculature. Pleural disease is the most common manifestation, occurring in 45–60% of patients. It may be asymptomatic, associated with pleuritic chest pain, or small to moderate pleural effusions.

'Shrinking lung syndrome' is a rare syndrome associated with lupus that is characterized by breathlessness, orthopnoea, and a characteristic radiological appearance of small lung volumes and elevated diaphragms (Figure 4.6). Reduced lung volumes are confirmed on pulmonary function testing and ultrasound screening of the diaphragm. It is thought to be a caused by diaphragmatic weakness.

Involvement of the lung parenchyma is rare in lupus, but the high frequency of pulmonary infections makes the exact prevalence hard to determine. Acute pneumonitis is described in <5% of patients. It is characterized by the rapid development of fever, cough, breathlessness, and hypoxia associated with patchy lung infiltrates on chest imaging. The mortality is up to 50%. Pulmonary haemorrhage is also rare and presents with a similar picture. Two-thirds of patients may have haemoptysis, but in those that do not, a blood stained bronchoalveolar lavage, elevated gas transfer on pulmonary function testing, and a fall in blood haemoglobin may help make the diagnosis. Mortality is high. The demonstration of immune-complex deposition within the alveolar wall and capillaries confirms that these serious manifestations are immune-mediated.

Chronic interstitial lung disease with lung fibrosis on CT scan is seen in approximately 10% of patients (Figure 4.7). It may be preceded by acute pneumonitis or develop in isolation. It is characterized by progressive breathlessness and sometimes a cough. Bilateral basal lung crackles are heard and a restrictive defect seen on pulmonary function testing. A non-specific interstitial pneumonia picture is more common on histology, but usual interstitial pneumonia is also seen.

Pulmonary hypertension develops in less than 15% of patients. It is usually mild and asymptomatic, detected on routine echocardiography or pulmonary function testing. Clinically overt pulmonary hypertension is found in <5% of unselected cases. When clinical symptoms do develop it is with progressive breathlessness and reduced exercise tolerance. Eventually signs of right heart failure develop. It is important to exclude recurrent thromboembolic disease as a cause. In the remaining cases the likely cause

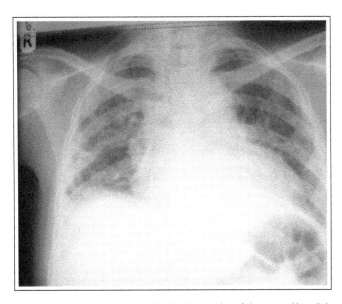

Figure 4.6 A chest radiograph of a patient with 'shrinking lung syndrome' characterized by radiological appearance of small lung volumes and elevated diaphragms as well as pulmonary fibrosis and cardiomegaly associated with pulmonary hypertension.

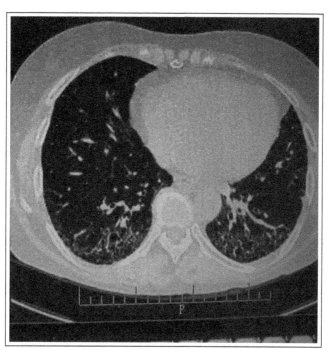

Figure 4.7 A CT scan of the lungs showing 'honey-combing' due to pulmonary fibrosis.

is a vasculopathy, similar to that seen in systemic sclerosis. Supporting this hypothesis is the high incidence of Raynaud's phenomenon and digital ulceration seen in patients with lupus-associated pulmonary hypertension.

The commonest cardiac manifestation of lupus is pericarditis, which develops in at least 50% of patients. Acute pericarditis typically presents with sharp anterior chest pain worse on lying down and relieved on sitting forwards. Severe cases may be accompanied by fever and tachycardia and a pericardial friction rub may be audible. Although unusual, cardiac tamponade can develop secondary to large pericardial effusions. Electrocardiographic changes can occur, including diffuse ST elevation and T wave abnormalities. Echocardiography will confirm the presence of an effusion and evaluate whether cardiac function is compromised.

Immune-mediated myocardial disease in lupus is rare. It is now well recognized that lupus per se is a potent independent risk factor for atheromatous vascular disease, similar to the risk associated with diabetes mellitus and small vessel ischaemia, and is probably the major factor contributing to progressive myocardial dysfunction. Acute immune-complex mediated myocarditis may present with signs of inflammation such as fever, tachycardia, and chest pain combined with evidence of ventricular dysfunction such as breathlessness, cough, orthopnoea, lower limb oedema, hepatic congestion, or frank pulmonary oedema. An electrocardiogram may reveal a number of non-specific abnormalities and/or arrhythmias (tachycardias or bradycardia including heart block). Endomyocardial biopsy has been the gold-standard diagnostic test and may help to distinguish viral myocarditis from lupus myocarditis, although cardiac MRI shows promise and may limit the need for invasive investigation to distinguish myocarditis from ischaemic heart disease.

Cardiac valve lesions are well described in patients with lupus, usually as an incidental finding. The archetypal cardiac valve lesions are small (<5 mm), non-infectious, verrucous lesions (Libman–Sachs or marantic endocarditis). They may be more common in patients with anti-phospholipid antibodies, but certainly not confined to this subgroup. Patients are usually asymptomatic, although a picture mimicking infectious endocarditis with fever, valvular dysfunction, and splinter haemorrhages can occur rarely. The course of valvular heart disease often does not reflect overall disease activity, adding to uncertainty over the aetiology.

Gastrointestinal disease

Abdominal pain is a relatively common cause of hospital admission in patients with SLE. Many cases are not directly lupus related, but may be related to medication (such as peptic ulceration or infection). Specific lupus-related causes are often not considered but include thrombotic disease (mesenteric, renal, and hepatic thrombosis), serositis (probably the most common presentation) or vasculitis presenting as pancreatitis, acalculous cholecystitis, or pseudo-obstruction. Lupus enteritis is an important and potentially life-threatening cause of acute abdomen but, as in common with many rarer features of lupus, it lacks a precise definition so interpreting prevalence statistics from the literature is difficult. Clinically the presentation can vary from an acute abdomen with vomiting and diarrhoea, pseudo-obstruction, or a protein-losing enteropathy. Previously considered as a vasculitis of visceral vessels, histological evaluation actually suggests that true vasculitis of the muscles in the intestinal wall is rare, and lupus enteritis is in most cases a direct inflammatory enteritis. There are no completely specific radiological features of lupus enteritis, but the typical CT appearance is of a multi-segmental, enhancing, bowel wall thickening with bowel dilatation, associated with prominent mesenteric vessels and attenuation and stranding of mesenteric fat. Lupus enteritis appears to be rare in the absence of other features of active disease. It should be noted that the SLEDAI disease activity instrument does not specifically score gastrointestinal (or ophthalmological) manifestations, unlike the BILAG 2004 index.

Although variably reported, abnormalities of liver function appear reasonably common, although often transient in lupus (25–50%), and three different mechanisms have been proposed to account for this. 1) Disease of the liver parenchyma directly caused by lupus—'lupus hepatitis'; 2) Overlap of lupus with another defined autoimmune liver disease such as autoimmune hepatitis or primary biliary cirrhosis; 3) co-occurrence of lupus with non-immune liver injury such as drug-induced or viral damage. Usually lupus hepatitis is an asymptomatic, steroid-responsive condition leading to a rise in transaminase enzymes in a patient with other manifestations of active lupus. Using this definition an incidence of lupus hepatitis of 9.3% was recently reported in a large cohort.

Ophthalmic

Lupus can affect any part of the visual system including the anterior and posterior segments of the eye and the optic nerve. The commonest manifestation is keratoconjunctivitis sicca, characterized by a reduction in the aqueous layer of the tear film and seen as a manifestation of secondary Sjögren's syndrome. Severity ranges from mild dryness with corneal epitheliopathy, to severe corneal ulceration. Involvement of the sclera is rare, reported in 2.4% of lupus patients. Most usual is episcleritis, which is a mild self-limiting condition causing discomfort and redness. Scleritis and anterior uveitis are rare in lupus.

Lupus retinopathy has been reported in up to 29% of lupus patients, although it appears to be becoming less frequent, perhaps as management of the disease in general improves. The commonest form of retinopathy is an immune-complex mediated microangiopathy characterized by cotton-wool spots, small intra-retinal haemorrhages, exudates, and microaneurysms. Mild retinopathy is usually asymptomatic, with more severe disease causing visual distortion/defects. Visual loss is rare. Neovascularization with secondary haemorrhage can occur. A true retinal vasculitis in which there is inflammation of retinal arterioles or venules is much less common and usually associated with the presence of anti-phospholipid antibodies. Severe visual loss secondary to central retinal vein or artery occlusion, vitreous haemorrhage, retinal ischaemia, or neovascularization can occur.

Optic nerve disease is rare in lupus. An optic neuritis, mimicking that seen in demyelinating disease can occur. It presents with a loss of visual acuity and has variable recovery. An optic neuropathy, thought to be due to a focal thrombotic event, can occur and presents with sudden visual loss. Small brainstem infarcts are also thought to underlie cranial nerve abnormalities seen in lupus, with 6th nerve palsies being the most common.

61

Conclusion

The range of disease manifestations seen in lupus means this condition presents a considerable challenge to the physician. It is important to consider objectively any new clinical feature as potentially due lupus, but equally important not to over-attribute every symptom as being lupus-related. Doing either risks harm as a result of missing important differential diagnoses or instituting unnecessarily aggressive immunosuppressive treatment regimens. It should be remembered that active lupus normally presents with several common clinical and immunological manifestations in addition to the occasional rare one. A single organ symptom out of proportion to the general picture of disease activity should always raise concern that lupus is not the answer.

Further reading

Disease activity

Yee CS, McElhone K, Teh LS, Gordon C. Assessment of disease activity and quality of life in systemic lupus erythematosus—New aspects. *Best Pract Res Clin Rheumatol* 2009;23:457–67.

Musculoskeletal

Ball EMA and Bell AL. Lupus arthritis: do we have a clinically useful classification? *Rheumatology* 2012;51:771–9.

Grossman JM. Lupus arthritis. *Best Prac Res Clin Rheumatol* 2009;23:495–506.

Cutaneous

Kuhn A and Landmann A. The classification and diagnosis of cutaneous lupus erythematosus. *J Autoimmunity* 2014;48–49:14–19.

Okon LG and Werth VP. Cutaneous lupus erythematosus. *Best Prac Res Clin Rheum.* 2013;27: 391–404.

Renal

Hahn BH, McMahon MA, Wilkinson A, et al. American College of Rheumatology guidelines for screening, treatment and management of lupus nephritis. *Arthritis Care Res* 2012;63:797–808.

KDIGO Kidney disease: improving global outcomes. Chapter 12: Lupus nephritis. In clinical practice guidelines for glomerulonephritis. *Kidney Int Suppl* 2012;2:221–32.

Haematological

Hepburn AL, Narat S and Mason JC. The management of peripheral blood cytopenias in systemic lupus erythematosus. *Rheumatology* 2010;49:2243–54.

Matta BN, Uthman I, Taher AT and Khamashta MA. The current understanding of diagnosis of antiphospholipid syndrome associated with systemic lupus erythematosus. *Expert Rev Clin Immunol* 2013; 9:659–68.

Ortel TL. Antiphospholipid syndrome: laboratory testing and diagnostic strategies. *Am J Hematol* 2012; 87suppl1:S75–81.

Vaulgarelis M, Kokori SI, Ioannidis JP, et al. Anaemia in systemic lupus erythematosus: Aetiological profile and the role of erythropoietin. *Ann Rheum Dis* 2000;59:217–22.

Neuropsychiatric

Bertsias GK, Ioannidis JPA, Aringer M et al. EULAR recommendations for the management of systemic lupus erythematosus with neuropsychiatric manifestations: report of a task force of the EULAR standing committee for clinical affairs. *Ann Rheum Dis* 2010;69:2074–82.

Hanley JG. Diagnosis and management of neuropsychiatric SLE. *Nat Rev Rheumatol* 2014;10:338–47.

Cardiorespiratory

Miner JJ and Kim AH. Cardiac manifestations of systemic lupus erythematosus. *Rheum Dis Clin North Am* 2014;40:51–60.

Mira-Avendano IC, and Abril A. Pulmonary manifestations of Sjogren's syndrome, systemic lupus erythematosus, and mixed connective tissue disease. *Rheum Dis Clin North Am.* 2015;41:263–77.

Gastrointestinal

Bessone F, Poles N and Roma MG. Challenge of liver disease in systemic lupus erythematosus: Clues for diagnosis and hints for pathogenesis. *World J Hepatol* 2014;6:394–409.

Hallegua DS and Wallace DJ. Gastrointestinal manifestations of systemic lupus erythematosus. *Curr Opin Rheum* 2000;12:379–85.

Janssens P, Amaud L, Galicier L, et al. Lupus enteritis: from clinical findings to therapeutic management. *Orphanet J Rare Dis* 2013;8:67.

Ophthalmological

Palejwala NV, Walia HS and Yeh S. Ocular manifestations of systemic lupus erythematosus: A review of the literature. *Autoimmune Dis* 2012. Epub: doi: 10.1155/2012/290898.

Papagiannuli E, Rhodes B, Wallace GR, et al. Systemic lupus erythematosus: an update for ophthalmologists. *Surv Ophthalmol* 2015 S0039-6257(15)00110-1 [pii]; doi: 10.1016/j.survophthal.2015.06.003.

Constitutional

Esposito S, Bosis S, Semino M and Rigante D. Infections and systemic lupus erythematosus. *Eur J Microbiol Infect Dis* 2014;33:1467–75.

Chapter 5

Laboratory tests and investigations

Anthony Isaacs and David Isenberg

Key points

- Basic haematological, biochemical, and immunological tests should be performed in the initial assessment of a patient suspected of having systemic lupus erythematosus (SLE).
- As a heterogeneous, multisystem disease, further investigations should be considered to confirm organ/system involvement and/or determine the extent of abnormality.
- A systems/organ-based approach is useful to identify the often protean manifestations.
- Long-term monitoring of lupus activity should be performed using specific laboratory testing, as well organ/system-based investigations where abnormalities have previously been identified.

63

Introduction

Investigations in patients with SLE serve several broad purposes: to assist in diagnosis, assess disease activity, distinguish disease subsets, identify end-organ damage, screen for associated autoimmune conditions, support treatment decisions, monitor side effects, judge response to treatment, and provide some idea about prognosis.

The initial investigations in SLE are aimed at determining the range of organ/system involvement and the extent of the immunological abnormalities (see Table 5.1). Follow-up tests focus on those biomarkers, notably anti-double stranded DNA antibodies (anti-dsDNA antibody) and complement component C3, which offer a guide to activity and tests of organ/system dysfunction where previous investigations have shown lupus involvement (see Table 5.2).

As SLE is a heterogeneous condition, we have used an organ-based approach to describe the use of investigations. This is divided into manifestations affecting the following systems: haematological, immunological, biochemical, renal, cardiovascular, pulmonary, gastroenterological, neurological, dermatological, and musculoskeletal.

Haematological

Haematological tests are essential in the assessment of SLE. They can be used to monitor disease activity, including response to treatment and complications of drug therapy, and to detect associated autoimmune conditions. The American College of Rheumatology

Table 5.1 Summary of the basic investigations for the initial assessment of a patient suspected to have lupus

Immunological	Organ/system	Consider also in certain situations
Anti-nuclear antibodies (ANA)	Full blood count (FBC)	Chest X-ray (CXR)
Extractible nuclear antigen (ENA)	Urea and electrolytes (U&Es)	Lung function
Rheumatoid factor	Erythrocyte sedimentation rate (ESR)	Electrocardiogram (ECG)
Anti-dsDNA antibody	C-reactive protein (CRP)	Neuropsychiatric testing
C3 and C4	Liver function tests (LFTs)	Organ imaging (eg, magnetic resonance imaging of the brain)
Anti-thyroid antibodies	Urine dipstick and protein-creatinine ratio (PCR)	
Coombs test	Blood pressure	
Coagulation		
Anti-cardiolipin antibodies		
Anti-β2-glycoprotein-1		
Lupus anticoagulant		

(ACR) SLE classification criteria recognize haematological involvement as: haemolytic anaemia with reticulocytosis; leucopenia $<4 \times 10^9/L$ on two occasions; lymphopenia $<1.5 \times 10^9/L$ on two occasions; and thrombocytopenia $<100 \times 10^9/L$ in the absence of an offending drug. Haematological involvement as defined by these criteria is present in around 60% of patients with SLE. The SLICC classification criteria for SLE provide an alternative classification, with similar haematological parameters, though lymphopenia is defined as $<1.0 \times 10^9/L$ and to meet the criteria, haematological abnormalities only need to be present on one occasion. Also a positive Coombs' test is deemed significant as a criterion in itself, but only in the absence of haemolysis. SLICC also differs from the ACR criteria through the inclusion of a wider range of cutaneous and neurological manifestations, nasal ulceration, non-scarring alopecia, and low complement (C3, C4, and CH50).

Full blood count

Anaemia

Anaemia is present in approximately 50% of patients.[1] The causes of anaemia in SLE can be divided into microcytic, normocytic, macrocytic, and haemolytic.[2]

A microcytic anaemia maybe a consequence of the anaemia of chronic disease; steroid- or non-steroidal anti-inflammatory drug (NSAID)-related peptic ulcer disease; dietary deficiency of iron; gastrointestinal blood loss; or menorrhagia. There

Table 5.2 Summary of basic investigations for monitoring disease activity in lupus

Immunological	Organ/system
C3 and C4	Full blood count (FBC)
Anti-double stranded DNA antibody (anti-dsDNA)	Urea and electrolytes (U&Es)
	Erythrocyte sedimentation rate (ESR)
	C-reactive protein (CRP)
	Liver function tests (LFTs)
	Urine dipstick
	Urine protein-creatinine ratio (PCR)
	Blood pressure

will be decreased serum iron, increased total iron binding capacity, microcytosis, and hypochromasia on the blood film. In some lupus populations, haemoglobinopathy maybe more prevalent, and testing should be considered in this context.

A normocytic anaemia can be due to myelosuppression from immunosuppressive medication; decreased erythropoietin levels if there is significant renal damage from lupus nephritis; macrophage activation syndrome (MAS); or acute bleeding in alveolar haemorrhage or in the context of autoimmune thrombocytopenia.

A macrocytic anaemia maybe as a result of immunosuppression (eg, azathioprine or methotrexate induced folate deficiency), or associated autoimmune diseases such as hypothyroidism, coeliac disease, or pernicious anaemia.

Autoimmune haemolytic anaemia due to SLE activity is demonstrated with fragments on blood film, an increased reticulocyte count, low haptoglobin, raised lactate dehydrogenase (LDH) and indirect bilirubin, and a positive Coombs test.

White cells

The prevalence of leucopenia in SLE is up to 66% at diagnosis. Lymphopenia prevalence is reported in up to 81%, which may represent active immune-mediated disease. Leucopenia from active SLE must be differentiated from drug side effects (eg, azathioprine, methotrexate, mycophenolate mofetil, or cyclophosphamide) or infection induced by the presence of a normal bone marrow.

Neutropenia may be seen in up to 50% of patients, as a consequence of immune-disease activity, medication, myelodysplasia, myelofibrosis, infection, or MAS. It may also be a normal variant in patients of African descent, independent of lupus disease activity.

Leucocytosis is invariably due to infection or as a result of steroid therapy.

Platelets (thrombocytopenia)

Thrombocytopenia in SLE has multiple potential aetiologies, and occurs in 10–20% of patients with SLE. It may be acute thrombocytopenia associated with major generalized disease activity; chronic mild thrombocytopenia most commonly associated with antiphospholipid antibodies; isolated idiopathic thrombocytopenic purpura (ITP) without other features of SLE (and may predate the diagnosis of lupus in 15%); Evan's syndrome; thrombotic thrombocytopenic purpura (rare disorder of small blood vessel thromboses resulting in microangiopathic haemolysis, thrombocytopenic purpura, fever, neurological symptoms, and renal failure), disseminated intravascular coagulation from sepsis; drug induced (eg, methotrexate, cyclophosphamide or azathioprine); or MAS.[3]

ESR

Erythrocyte sedimentation rate (ESR) measures the distance in millimetres that red cells fall in 1 hour. It is a variably useful marker of disease activity in SLE.

Coagulation defects

There may be a prolonged activated partial thromboplastin time (APTT) if lupus anticoagulant is present, as it interacts with the phospholipids in the assay.

Immunological

Complement

Complement is crucial in clearance of immune complexes.[4] Homozygous, hereditary deficiency of each of the classical pathway components (C1q, C1r, C1s, C4, and C2) are associated with an increased susceptibility to a lupus-like illness but are rare in clinical practice.

SLE has also been associated with acquired complement deficiency states, particularly in patients with reduced concentrations of C2 and C4 caused by the effects of inherited C1 inhibitor deficiency. The presence of C3 nephritic factor autoantibody, which causes C3 consumption, has also been associated with the presence of SLE.

During periods of active disease serum complement is reduced. Typically, concentrations of the classical pathway components (C1q, C2, C4) are low and, especially in patients with severe disease, are often accompanied by a reduction in C3 concentration. Therefore, regular monitoring of the C3 concentration is a key tool, as a falling C3 concentration maybe a predictor of an impending disease flare. The new SLICC classification has included a low serum C3 as a criterion (unlike the revised ACR criteria). Breakdown products of C3 and C4 (eg, C3d and C4d) are often high in active disease, but lack of commercial kits means they are rarely tested for.

SLE also causes activation and consumption of C1q. It has been demonstrated that increases in anti-C1q antibody titres precede lupus nephritis in some, but not all patients.

Antinuclear antibodies

Antinuclear antibodies (ANA) are present in >95% of patients with SLE. They are immunoglobulins, usually IgG, that bind to antigens that are expressed in the nucleus of cells. Immunofluorescence using murine liver or kidney cells, or a human epithelial line (Hep-2 cells), has classically been used to detect them; although more rapid automated methods are now being widely introduced. A titre of 1:80 is regarded as weak positive, though may still represent autoimmune rheumatic disease and must be interpreted in the clinical context. In the elderly, or in infection states, they have a low positive predictive value, whereas a titre well over 1:640 or stronger would be regarded as significant and may indicate the presence of SLE or an autoimmune disease. ANA testing in SLE has an overall sensitivity of around 95%, and specificity 50%. It can also be positive in autoimmune liver or thyroid disease, transiently in infection, rheumatoid arthritis, Sjogren's' syndrome, polymyositis/dermatomyositis, systemic sclerosis, drug-induced lupus erythematous, or usually in low titre in up to 30% of the normal population.

There are a number of ANA staining patterns that are linked to the precise antigen target (see Figures 5.1 and 5.2).[5]

Double stranded DNA

Anti-double stranded DNA antibodies (dsDNA) are often raised in SLE and are associated most strongly with proliferative lupus nephritis. They have a sensitivity of approximately 55% and specificity of approximately 95% in SLE. High concentrations may indicate disease activity, and a rising concentration on serial measurements may predict a flare. Thus they are useful for clinical monitoring, and may become undetectable when disease is in remission. They are tested by an enzyme-linked immunosorbent assay (ELISA); immunofluorescence with *Crithidia luciliae* (a haemoflagellated organism); or the Farr test (Farr immunoprecipitation assays detecting high affinity antibodies) (see Figure 5.3). In practice, as the Farr assay is radioactively-dependent, few labs undertake this routinely. Anti-dsDNA antibodies can be seen transiently due to infection or drug-induced SLE but they are usually considered a reliable marker of SLE, although they are only present in about 55–60% of patients.

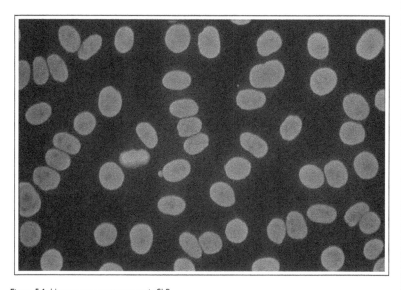

Figure 5.1 Homogenous pattern seen in SLE.

Morrow J, Nelson L, Watts R, Isenberg DA. Autoimmune Rheumatic Disease 2nd Edition (1999), by permission of Oxford University Press.

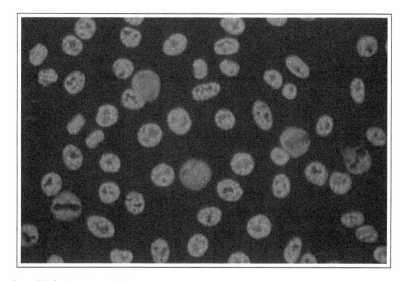

Figure 5.2 Speckled: A speckled pattern seen in overlap conditions with Sjogren's syndrome, systemic sclerosis, and undifferentiated autoimmune rheumatic disease.

Morrow J, Nelson L, Watts R, Isenberg DA. Autoimmune Rheumatic Disease 2nd Edition (1999), by permission of Oxford University Press.

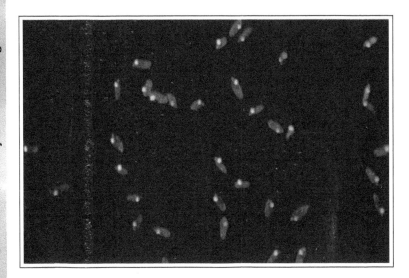

Figure 5.3 Crithidia dsDNA.

Morrow J, Nelson L, Watts R, Isenberg DA. Autoimmune Rheumatic Disease 2nd Edition (1999), by permission of Oxford University Press.

Extractable nuclear antigens

Antibodies to the extractable nuclear antigens (ENAs) Ro, La, and Smith (Sm), and to ribonucleoprotein (RNP), are often tested by Immunoblot or ELISA. In SLE, Anti-Ro antibodies are present in 30–40% of patients, and anti-La antibodies present in 10–15%, suggesting an overlap with Sjogren's syndrome. In pregnant lupus patients who are positive for Ro or La, there is a 5–10% risk of neonatal lupus, which may cause a photosensitive rash developing up to 6 months after birth (usually resolving within 3 months) and a 1–2% risk of congenital complete heart block (which is invariably permanent). Anti-Sm is present in 30% of Afro-Caribbean patients and 10% of Caucasians. Anti-RNP is positive in 30–40% of patients and may be linked to overlap conditions including myositis. Anti-centromere antibodies are often found in limited cutaneous systemic sclerosis and can be positive in overlap syndromes with SLE.

Anti-histone antibodies

These are present in 95% of drug-induced SLE but also in around 50% SLE. IgM or IgG antibodies can be detected by Immunoblot or ELISA.

Anti-nucleosome

This is an immunoassay that is commercially available, but rather expensive. Meta-analysis reveals they have a sensitivity of 61% and specificity of 94% which may be better than testing for anti-dsDNA antibodies. They may also be a good marker of disease activity.

Rheumatoid factor

Rheumatoid factors are immunoglobulins (IgM, IgG, or IgA) that bind to the constant region (Fc portion) of immunoglobulin G (IgG). It is positive in about 25% of patients with SLE and may represent an overlap with rheumatoid arthritis (rhupus).

Anti-cyclic citrullinated peptide antibodies

These immunoglobulins are rarely found in SLE patients and may be associated with arthritis.

Antiphospholipid antibodies

Antiphospholipid antibodies maybe present in association with SLE, and suggest a potential predisposition to thrombosis and maternal pregnancy morbidity. There are three main antibody tests, antiocardiolipin antibody, lupus anticoagulant, and anti-β2-glycoprotein-1 antibody. The more of these antibodies that are positive, the greater the risk is of clinical events.

Anticardiolipin antibody

IgG and IgM anticardiolipin antibodies are usually detected by ELISA, and are found in 30–40% of SLE patients. The presence of IgG anticardiolipin antibodies, especially in high titre, is more significant in terms of risk of events. These antibodies may be detectable in SLE with antiphospholipid syndrome (APS), primary APS, or infection.

Lupus anticoagulant

Lupus anticoagulant is a haematological, not an immunological test, but is presented in this section to accompany the other antiphospholipid syndrome investigations. A positive test result for lupus anticoagulant is a strong predictor of thrombotic events or pregnancy morbidity. It can be positive in APS associated with SLE, primary APS, and infection. It is suspected with a prolonged APTT, which does not correct after mixing patient plasma with normal plasma (this is confirmed when patients plasma is mixed with a high phospholipid load in the form of platelets, which corrects the prolonged APTT).

Anti-β2-glycoprotein-1 antibody

Autoantibodies to β2-glycoprotein-1 are detected by immunoassays. IgG and IgM can be detected. This can be positive in SLE with APS, primary APS, or following thrombosis or infection.

Biochemical

Inflammatory markers (CRP)

C-reactive protein (CRP) is often normal in active SLE, and this phenomenon appears to be unique to SLE. However, CRP does rise in specific circumstances such as severe arthritis, serositis with effusions and, importantly, with infection.

Liver function

Coexistent autoimmune liver disease causing a raised alanine aminotransferase (ALT) or aspartate aminotransferase (AST) occurs in approximately 5% of patients with SLE. A transaminitis can also be caused by liver toxicity from many drugs, particularly immunosuppressive drugs and NSAIDs. Transaminitis may also be due to overlap myositis, as these enzymes are also produced in the skeletal muscle, and so the creatine kinase (CK) should be tested. It is important to test for viral hepatitis B and C prior to immunosuppression, especially in the context of raised transaminases, and also to consider cytomegalovirus (CMV) testing when on immunosuppressive therapy.

Alkaline phosphatase (ALP) can rise as an acute phase marker with inflammation, liver disease from hepatotoxins, or SLE, or it may represent metabolic bone disease with vitamin D deficiency. A gamma-glutamyl transferase (GGT) or ALP isoenzymes test can be used to differentiate from liver/biliary sources.

A low serum albumin is usually the consequence of lupus nephritis with significant proteinuria, or much less frequently can be as a result of active autoimmune liver disease. Sepsis, liver disease, and protein-losing enteropathy can also result in hypoalbuminaemia.

Bone profile and vitamin D

Lupus patients are often advised to avoid exposure to sunlight as their disease may be exacerbated. However, this advice may lead to low levels of vitamin D. In order to preserve bone strength it is important to maintain adequate levels of calcium, phosphate, and vitamin D. Osteoporosis is a particular problem in those on long term prednisolone (>6 mg/day), and dual-energy X-ray absorptiometry (DXA) should be performed.

Muscle enzymes

Creatine kinase (CK) concentration will be raised in overlap syndromes with myositis, present in around 4% of patients. CK should be tested in the presence of a transaminitis as this may be due to concomitant muscle disease. Serum aldolase and lactate dehydrogenase (LDH) may also be elevated. Electromyography can be performed to determine if there is a myopathy, even if the muscle enzymes are not elevated. A muscle biopsy is the definitive test in assessing for a myositis.

Thyroid

Autoimmune diseases are a family, and autoimmune thyroid disease is well recognized in lupus patients. Approximately 8% are hypothyroid and 1–2% hyperthyroid. Autoimmune thyroid disease may be more prevalent in patients with coexistent Sjogren's' syndrome. Thyroglobulin and thyroid peroxidase antibodies are detected frequently in around 10–15%, even in the absence of clinical disease. This situation may predict those at risk in the future, and so occasional testing of thyroxine (T4) and thyroid stimulating hormone (TSH) are advised, especially if the patient reports new onset fatigue, or if they may be pregnant.

Renal

Urinalysis is one of the most vital tests in detecting renal involvement, in addition to blood urea, creatinine, estimated glomerular filtration rate (eGFR), and serum albumin levels. Renal involvement can be detected initially with urine dipstick demonstration of haematuria and protein. This is very important as detection of proteinuria and haematuria may antedate renal function impairment. Further evidence is the presence of red cell casts in the urine, which is highly suggestive of glomerular damage from a glomerular-based process. Red cell casts are also seen in other conditions such as vasculitis and Goodpasture's syndrome.

Quantification of urinary protein concentration should be performed. This historically involved a 24-hour urine protein collection. Nephrotic range proteinuria is defined as urinary excretion of above 3 g/day. A spot urine protein/creatinine ratio is now felt to be adequate because of its convenience, and removal of the collection error that can occur with a 24-hour sample. A urine protein/creatinine ratio exceeding 50 mg/mmol is felt to be significant. Nephrotic range proteinuria is approximately equivalent to 300 mg/mmol. There is a broad differential diagnosis for proteinuria including NSAID-induced interstitial nephritis and diabetes mellitus (reported in 2–6% of SLE patients) which may need to be considered.

Table 5.3 ISN/RPS 2003 classification of lupus nephritis (LN)	
Class I	Minimal mesangial LN
Class II	Mesangial proliferative LN
Class III	Focal LN* (<50% of glomeruli)
	III (A): active lesions
	III (A/C): active and chronic lesions
	III (C): chronic lesions
Class IV	Diffuse LN* (≥50% of glomeruli)
	Diffuse segmental (IV-S) or global (IV-G) LN
	IV (A): active lesions
	IV (A/C): active and chronic lesions
	IV (C): chronic lesions
Class V	Membranous LN
Class VI	Advanced sclerosing LN
	(≥90% globally sclerosed glomeruli without residual activity)

ISN/RPS 2003 classification.

Renal biopsy should be considered for all cases of active lupus nephritis prior to treatment, and is rarely contraindicated. It is also useful in relapsing or refractory cases of lupus nephritis. The main aim of biopsy is to classify the disease and its activity in order to guide treatment decisions. It may also offer prognostic information.

The different subtypes of lupus nephritis are described by the ISN/RPS 2003 classification (see Table 5.3) and accompanying biopsy picture (Figure 5.4 (see colour version on inside cover)).

Cardiovascular

Cardiac manifestations of SLE include myocarditis, pericarditis, and Libman–Sacks endocarditis.

Cardiac enzymes

Cardiac enzymes including troponin can be elevated in the presence of a lupus myocarditis.

Electrocardiogram (ECG)

The electrocardiogram typically shows low voltage complexes, widespread saddle-shaped ST elevation, or PR depression in pericarditis with a pericardial effusion. Myocarditis may cause a sinus tachycardia, conduction blocks, or overt arrhythmias.

Echocardiography

A transthoracic echocardiogram can reveal a pericardial effusion in acute pericarditis. In SLE this is rarely clinically significant enough to cause tamponade. In myocarditis there may be cardiomegaly or biventricular failure. Rarely, thickening of the aortic or mitral valve, or overt vegetations are found in Libman–Sacks endocarditis due to SLE or

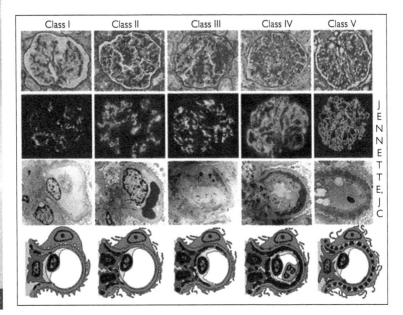

Figure 5.4 Lupus nephritis biopsy findings. (See colour version on inside cover.)
J. Charles Jennette, MD. Courtesy of www.unckidneycenter.org

anti-phospholipid syndrome (APS), and are more commonly seen post-mortem suggesting a significant volume of subclinical disease. Valvular lesions can be further characterized with transoesophageal echocardiography. A raised right ventricular systolic pressure may be found, suggestive of pulmonary arterial hypertension (PAH), pulmonary embolism in APS, or SLE parenchymal lung disease.

Cardiac magnetic resonance imaging (MRI)

Cardiac MRI has emerged as an essential non-invasive assessment of myocarditis. The typical appearance is enhancement on T2 weighted images without fat saturation suggestive of myocardial inflammation. A right ventricular endomyocardial biopsy can confirm lupus myocarditis if the aetiology is unclear.

Cardiovascular risk

The University of Pittsburgh Medical Center study found that women with SLE aged 35–44 years are over 50-times more likely to have a myocardial infarction compared with women of a similar age. Therefore checking and managing conventional cardiovascular risk factors is important in patient follow-up, including measurement of blood pressure, smoking cessation, lowering of serum lipids, HBA1c, and glucose.

Pulmonary

There are numerous pulmonary manifestations of SLE, often requiring several investigations.

Pulmonary function testing

Pulmonary function testing is useful in the assessment of interstitial lung disease. This is considered to be present when there is a reduction in forced expiratory volume in one second (FEV_1) and forced vital capacity (FVC) with a normal or increased FEV_1/FVC ratio. A low FVC and diffusion capacity for carbon monoxide (DL_{CO}) may suggest interstitial lung disease (ILD) or a pneumonitis. The DL_{CO} is raised in the context of pulmonary haemorrhage, due to haemoglobin in the alveolar spaces. Reduced lung volumes and diffusion capacity with a restrictive pattern on spirometry, along with chest radiographic evidence of small volume lung space and raised hemi-diaphragms is suggestive of shrinking lung syndrome.

Plain chest radiographs

Plain chest radiographs may reveal reticulonodular changes due to ILD. An organizing pneumonia often presents with patchy consolidation. Pneumonia as a consequence of immunosuppression is a frequent concern. Diffuse alveolar shadowing can be caused by pulmonary haemorrhage or lupus pneumonitis (associated with Ro antibody). Serositis can cause pleural effusions which are often bilateral. A pleural effusion or wedge-shaped infarct can be seen with a pulmonary embolism. In lupus myocarditis, the plain film may show cardiomegaly, alveolar oedema, pleural effusions, upper lobe vein diversion, and fluid in the horizontal fissure. The finding of hilar lymphadenopathy raises the question of associated Kikuchi' disease or lymphoma, or carcinoma of the lung which is more common in lupus patients who smoke. In the shrinking lung syndrome, there are often raised hemidiaphragms with small volume lungs (see Figure 4.6).

All of these findings are better delineated on CT imaging of the chest.

Bronchoscopy +/− biopsy and bronchoalveolar lavage

Bronchoscopy +/− biopsy and bronchoalveolar lavage (BAL) sent for cell count, bacterial, viral and fungal culture, and cytology is valuable in the assessment of lung disease. This helps to establish the diagnosis, and to exclude the more common opportunistic organisms such as tuberculosis and other atypical mycobacteria, CMV, *Pneumocystis jirovecii*, *Aspergillus*, and *Nocardia*. In the presence of pneumonitis, biopsy can reveal oedema, hyaline membrane formation, and perivascular inflammation. Pulmonary haemorrhage may be visible, or detected on BAL with haemosiderin-laden macrophages, or with biopsy evidence of capillaritis with immune complexes or bland haemorrhage.

Computerized tomographic pulmonary angiography

Computerized tomographic pulmonary angiography (CTPA) may reveal pulmonary embolism, especially in the context of coexistent APS.

Right heart catheterization

Right-sided heart catheterization is performed to investigate suspected pulmonary arterial hypertension after other causes such as lung disease and pulmonary embolism have been excluded. This investigation may rarely reveal pre-capillary pulmonary arterial hypertension (mean pulmonary arterial pressure ≥25 mmHg and pulmonary wedge pressure of <15 mmHg). Pulmonary arterial hypertension is more common in patients with antiphospholipid antibodies, Raynaud's and overlap syndromes, but it is present in <5% of SLE patients overall.

Pleural, pericardial fluid analysis

Aspiration of pericardial or pleural fluid can be analysed for features of SLE. Lupus serositis will result in an exudative effusion, positive antinuclear antibody, low complement, high lactate dehydrogenase, and normal glucose (low in rheumatoid arthritis and empyema). The cell count often reveals a moderately elevated white cell count, predominantly polymorphs in the early SLE, and lymphocytes in later disease.

Gastrointestinal

Mesenteric vasculitis is rare is patients with SLE occurring in <5%. An abdominal CT may show bowel thickening with the target sign (abnormal bowel wall enhancement), mesenteric oedema, and ascites. A mesenteric angiogram will reveal microaneurysms.

Neurological

Electromyography

Electromyography (EMG) is used to identify a myopathy, more common in overlap dermatomyositis or polymyositis. The classical findings of an autoimmune myositis are spontaneous positive sharp waves; polyphasic potentials of short duration and low amplitude; high frequency repetitive discharges; and fibrillation at rest. The possibility of a steroid or medication-induced myopathy should be considered, particularly if the findings of the EMG are non-inflammatory. Muscle biopsy can be performed if there is diagnostic doubt and remains the gold standard test. In an autoimmune myositis there is often vascular and perivascular inflammation.

Nerve conduction studies

A nerve conduction study may be used to detect suspected mononeuritis multiplex, symmetrical polyneuropathy, or an acute demyelinating polyradiculopathy. If expertise is available, nerve conduction studies may be used to identify cranial nerve involvement. A nerve biopsy is not always helpful as there are usually non-specific findings.

Lumbar puncture

This is essential in the investigation of suspected central nervous system (CNS) lupus, and to exclude CNS infection. This is performed in patients with a suspected encephalopathy, stroke, seizures, or transverse myelitis. Cerebrospinal fluid (CSF) findings are often of a normal white and red cell count, culture, and glucose, but with a raised protein concentration. The protein concentration, however, may also be normal, and a raised lymphocyte count or low glucose may be seen, making it difficult to differentiate from infection (eg, tuberculosis or viruses). Specific CSF and serum oligoclonal bands may be positive, suggestive of CNS inflammation.

Magnetic resonance imaging

Magnetic resonance imaging of the brain or spinal cord is widely used in the assessment of CNS lupus. An MRI of the spine can be used also to identify transverse myelitis, and to exclude compressive lesions.

MRI of the brain is used to assess lupus cerebritis, which involves the small blood vessels. Subtle abnormalities can include multiple small T2-signal white matter lesions or vague areas of patchy cortical or subcortical abnormality, although the imaging can also be completely normal. SLE is more likely than MS radiologically when lesions do not involve the periventricular white matter, and these diseases are very rarely concomitant (<1% of SLE patients). Conventional angiography of the cerebral vessels is unlikely to demonstrate lupus lesions due to the small vessel size, unlike other types of CNS vasculitis.

Brain biopsy

A brain biopsy can be performed to exclude neoplastic disease or opportunistic infection that cannot be differentiated clinically from CNS lupus. In lupus cerebritis the pathological findings are of a small vessel vasculopathy.

Electroencephalogram (EEG)

This can be useful in identifying seizure activity in challenging cases. It can also be used to assess risk of seizure recurrence. An active spike focus particularly with multiple loci, frequent discharges, or localization to the frontotemporal region suggests a likely recurrence of seizures after discontinuing anticonvulsant therapy.

Dermatological

Skin manifestations of lupus are diverse.[6] They can occur in the context of systemic lupus, or solely as a dermatological condition in cutaneous lupus without systemic disease. Skin biopsy for histology, often with immunofluorescence, is frequently necessary for diagnosis and exclusion of non-lupus pathology.

The subtypes of cutaneous lupus can be divided as shown in Table 5.4.

The lupus band test

The lupus band test is a useful tool that can be used to confirm lupus lesions, differentiate systemic lupus erythematous from cutaneous lupus, and exclude other cutaneous conditions.[7] It involves direct immunofluorescence to assess for the presence of immunoglobulins and complement at the dermo-epidermal junction.

Lupus arthropathy imaging

Imaging has been fundamental in developing a greater understanding of lupus arthropathy, as well as differentiating it from overlapping erosive arthropathies.[8,9] Imaging is useful also as a research tool in objectively assessing joint inflammation and damage. The main imaging modalities used are plain film, ultrasound, and MRI. The optimal imaging method to identify subclinical pathology not seen on plain radiographs has yet to be established between MRI and ultrasound.

Plain film

The classical changes of Jaccoud's arthropathy, with ulnar deviation of the 2nd to 5th digits and subluxation of metacarpophalangeal joints, are seen on plain radiographs. In this context "hook-shaped erosions" in the metacarpal heads of the hands and feet, said to be a consequence of bone trauma due to misplaced tendon sheaths are occasionally present. The erosive changes of 'rhupus' can be seen also affecting the wrists, metacarpophalangeal joints, and proximal interphalangeal joints, with periarticular

Table 5.4 Subtypes of cutaneous lupus	
SLE	Immune deposits at the dermal-epidermal junction Slight to absent epidermal atrophy Basement membrane zone of normal thickness No follicular plugging Prominent papillary dermal oedema and reticular mucin accumulation
Subacute cutaneous lupus	Prominent suprabasilar exocytosis of lymphocytes Dyskeratosis extending into the upper spinous layers Prominent epidermal atrophy Follicular plugging or basement membrane thickening zone minimal or absent Mild to moderate mononuclear cell infiltrate confined to the superficial dermis
Discoid lupus erythematous	Lymphocyte rich interface dermatitis Less epidermal atrophy than subacute cutaneous lupus; sometimes acanthosis Prominent follicular hyperkeratosis Dense superficial and deep perivascular and periadnexal infiltrates Prominent follicular degeneration Dermal fibrosis
Leucocytoclastic vasculitis	Vascular and perivascular infiltration of polymorphonuclear leucocytes with fragmentation of neutrophils, extravasation of erythrocytes, and fibrinoid necrosis of the vessel walls
Urticarial vasculitis	Leucocytoclasia, erythrocyte extravasation, neutrophil invasion of vessel walls, and minimal fibrin deposition
Lymphocytic vasculitis	Lymphocyte infiltration involving and surrounding the small vessel walls of the dermis with fibrin deposition in the vessel walls This is more common if coexistent cryofibrinogenaemia or lupus anticoagulant
Livedo reticularis	Segmental hyalinizing vascular involvement of thickened dermal blood vessels, endothelial proliferation, and focal thrombosis without nuclear dust
Bullous lupus erythematous	Subepidermal blisters with dermal inflammation characterized by neutrophilic papillary abscesses Neutrophilic interface dermatitis Histiocytes
Lupus Profundus	Subcutaneous fat lobules infiltrated with lymphocytes, histiocytes, and plasma cells within interposed zone of granular necrobiotic alteration There may also be endothelial necrosis, segmental deposits of fibrin, occlusive luminal thrombi of interstitial capillaries, and venules
Chillblain lupus	Vacuolar interface dermatitis Lymphocytic vascular reaction involving venules within the dermis Mural and luminal fibrin deposition within reticular dermal vessels
Drug induced lupus	In drug-induced SLE there is a cell-poor vacuolopathic lymphocytic interface injury pattern, with superficial disposition of the infiltrate, and absent keratotic follicular plugging or basement membrane zone thickening In drug-induced cutaneous lupus the findings are similar to SCLE but with deeper perivascular extension of the infiltrate

Crowson AN, Magro C. The cutaneous pathology of lupus erythematosus: a review. J Cutan Pathol. 2001; 28:1–23, Wiley.

osteopenia and joint space narrowing. About 4% of patients with SLE have concomitant rheumatoid arthritis.

Ultrasound

This can identify joint effusions with synovitis and neovascularity in active joint inflammation. Erosive changes are demonstrated and appear to be more common than previously expected. There also is a higher than anticipated frequency of tenosynovitis and tendon thickening.

Magnetic resonance imaging

Similarly to ultrasound, this successfully demonstrates synovitis, erosions, and tenosynovitis. It is less operator dependent than ultrasound scanning. Erosions on MRI in SLE have been reported in up to 93% at the wrist, and 61% in the metacarpophalangeal joints. This interestingly appears to be independent of rhupus, with the majority of these patients being both rheumatoid factor and anti-cyclic citrullinated peptide antibody negative.

References

1. Giannouli S, Voulgarelis M, Ziakas PD, Tzioufas AG. Anaemia in systemic lupus erythematosus: from pathophysiology to clinical assessment. *Ann Rheum Dis* 2006;65:144.

2. Manson JJ, Isenberg DA, Chambers S, Shipley ME, Merrill JT. *Rapid review of rheumatology and musculoskeletal disorders* CRC Press, Florida, USA. 2014.

3. Keeling DM, Isenberg DA. Haematological manifestations of systemic lupus erythematosus. *Blood Rev* 1993;7:199–207.

4. Pickering MC, Walpaort MJ. Links between complement abnormalities and systemic lupus erythematosus. *Rheumatology* 2000;39:133.

5. Morrow J, Nelson L, Watts R, Isenberg DA. *Autoimmune rheumatic disease* 2nd Ed. Oxford University Press, Oxford, UK. 1999. Fig 2.11 (p 33).

6. Crowson AN, Magro C. The cutaneous pathology of lupus erythematosus: a review. *J Cutan Pathol* 2001;28:1–23.

7. Reich A. Marcinow K, Bialynicki-Birula R. The lupus band test in systemic lupus erythematous patients. *Ther Clin Risk Manag* 2011;7:27–32.

8. Ball EM, Tan AL, Fukuba E, et al. A study of erosive phenotypes in lupus arthritis using magnetic resonance imaging and anti-citrullinated protein antibody, anti-RA33 and RF autoantibody status. *Rheumatology* (Oxford). 2014;53:1835–43.

9. Ball EM, Bell AL. Lupus arthritis: do we have a clinically useful classification? *Rheumatology* (Oxford). 2012;51:771–9.

Chapter 6

Conventional treatments in systemic lupus erythematosus

Anisur Rahman

> ### Key points
>
> - It is important to remember non-drug interventions that can help in the management of patients with SLE; these include education, sun-protection, and stopping smoking.
> - Milder forms of SLE, such as rash, fatigue, and hair loss, are not life-threatening but may have a major impact on quality of life.
> - Many patients with SLE do not require immunosuppression for long periods; their clinical features can be managed with symptomatic treatment such as analgesics and anti-inflammatory drugs.
> - There is good evidence that long-term treatment with oral antimalarial medication (most commonly hydroxychloroquine) should be recommended for patients with SLE as it improves long-term health outcomes.
> - Flares of joint pain, pericarditis, or pleurisy in patients with SLE can be treated with short courses of oral corticosteroids or intramuscular injections of depot corticosteroid preparations (such as methylprednisolone).
> - Induction of remission in patients with lupus nephritis can be achieved by treatment with high dose corticosteroids plus either oral mycophenolate or the Euro-Lupus low-dose intravenous cyclophosphamide regimen.
> - Remission of lupus nephritis is usually maintained by treatment with low-dose oral corticosteroids plus either oral mycophenolate or oral azathioprine.
> - Severe non-renal forms of SLE include neuropsychiatric lupus, severe anaemia, or thrombocytopenia, and lupus mesenteric vasculitis. The mainstay of treatment for all these is high-dose corticosteroids (oral or intravenous) with immunosuppressants such as mycophenolate or cyclophosphamide being used in refractory or severe cases.

Introduction

Imagine that you yourself were a patient just diagnosed with systemic lupus erythematosus (SLE) and that you had no medical knowledge. What would you want to know? What would be your fears and concerns? What would you want from your healthcare team? This chapter will look at the conventional management of SLE through the prism of the patient's expectations and will thus show how these questions may be addressed using conventional management strategies and therapies. Chapter 7 will address the place of the newer biologic therapies in the management of SLE.

What is SLE, and what effect will it have on my life?

SLE is a rare condition with a prevalence of about one in 1000 people in the UK in 2012.[1] This means that most people diagnosed with the disease will have no knowledge of it. Many may never have heard of it. SLE is 9–10 times more common in women than in men and tends to present under the age of 40. Thus our hypothetical newly-diagnosed patient is most likely to be a young woman who has gone from expecting to enjoy good health for many years to being a 'patient' with a chronic disease. This alone may be frightening and very upsetting for many patients. Looking up 'lupus' on the internet will rapidly produce a long list of serious complications and symptoms. Many of these may never affect the individual patient or may be easily treatable. In other words, it is important both at the time of diagnosis and in later consultations to be aware of the patient's beliefs and fears about the disease and to provide accurate information. There are good booklets from organizations such as Arthritis Research UK, LUPUS UK, and the Lupus Foundation of America which can be very helpful. Clinical nurse specialists can play a very valuable role in providing information and reassurance to patients. In some cases, the involvement of a psychologist may also help. These are generally cases in which patients have suffered long-term severe forms of lupus and/or where many different treatments have been tried and failed. The disease may have led to severe difficulties in maintaining education, employment, and/or family life. Psychological input will not resolve these problems but may help patients to find ways of improving their quality of life.

An obvious question for many patients is, 'will having lupus shorten my life?' Most textbooks and reviews about SLE stress the dramatic improvements in life expectancy over the last 50 years, from a 50% 5-year survival in the 1950s, to 80% 15-year survival in the 1990s.[2] A patient in their mid-20s however, could interpret that same figure as a one in five chance of dying by the age of 40. In fact, for most patients with mild disease, that early death would be very unlikely to happen; patients who die at a young age generally have severe lupus from early on in the disease. For most patients seen in a lupus clinic, therefore, a reasonable aim of treatment is to maintain a normal quality of life and normal life expectancy using medication. A particular issue relevant to young women with SLE is the potential effect on their chances of having a successful pregnancy. This will be addressed in more detail in Chapter 9 (Management of special situations in SLE).

In summary, SLE cannot be cured but it can be controlled. A patient diagnosed with SLE will likely always have SLE—although in some cases it may become quiescent. It is important to stress the importance of regular follow-up in a specialist centre where both symptoms and blood tests can be monitored, in order to recognize flares of the disease early, and treat them expeditiously.

What can I do to help myself?

It is important not to forget simple, lifestyle advice for patients with SLE. The most important thing of all is to protect oneself from ultraviolet solar radiation. The rash of

Table 6.1 Non-drug interventions to remember in managing patients with SLE	
Intervention	**Importance**
Education—use booklets	Reduces fear, increases knowledge, establishes expectations for treatment
Sun-protection—avoid strong sunlight and use sunblock	Reduces flares, especially in skin
Stop smoking	Improves cutaneous lupus. Reduces cardiovascular disease risk
Regular moderate exercise	May reduce cardiovascular disease risk and fatigue
Referral to clinical nurse specialist	Information, discussion of beliefs and concerns
Psychologist	Some patients with disease-related anxiety or severe effects of disease on lifestyle may benefit

SLE is often photosensitive, even in dark-skinned people; indeed photosensitivity is one of the American College of Rheumatology classification criteria for SLE.[3] Some patients suffer flares of systemic symptoms such as joint pain and tiredness as well as increased rash after exposure to the sun. Thus, in the summer and particularly on holidays in sunny places, patients should be advised to stay in the shade and use high protection factor sun-block.

Most studies have shown that between 10 and 20% of patients with SLE smoke. There are a number of good reasons why they should stop. Smoking increases the severity of skin disease in lupus and also increases the risk of developing cardiovascular disease. The prospect of heart attacks or strokes seems a remote one to many patients with SLE, given that they are young women with low baseline risk of these events. However, research has shown that, in the long-term, having lupus is itself an independent risk factor for developing cardiovascular disease so that reducing modifiable cardiovascular risk factors such as smoking is highly advisable.[4] In the 30–40% of patients of patients with SLE who have serum antiphospholipid antibodies, it is important to stop smoking to reduce the risk of developing venous thrombosis.

There is no secure evidence base for recommending particular forms of diet in patients with SLE. A balanced healthy diet is advisable and some older studies suggested that diets low in saturated fats and/or supplemented with fish oils could be beneficial for some patients. Patients taking corticosteroids may particularly find that they need to control their diet in order to avoid becoming overweight. Regular exercise is recommended, though many patients may find this difficult due to joint pain and fatigue. A randomized controlled trial from Tench et al. showed that patients with SLE who exercised regularly felt less fatigued than those who did not, but that it was difficult for patients to maintain the exercise regime after the trial had finished.[5]

Table 6.1 summarizes the non-drug measures that can be helpful in managing patients with SLE

Management of mild SLE: What medications can help my everyday symptoms?

The most common symptoms of SLE are rash, mouth ulcers, hair loss, joint pain, and fatigue. Most patients experience some or all of these symptoms at some stage and some suffer them every day. In most cases they can be managed and controlled (though not always eradicated) without the use of systemic corticosteroids or immunosuppressants. Nevertheless, it is important to remember that while these symptoms are not life-threatening they may have significant effects on the patient's lifestyle. Many patients with SLE find the effects of the disease on their appearance—such as bald patches, facial rash, and weight gain and hirsutism due to corticosteroids—particularly upsetting.

Skin and hair

Apart from sun-protection and stopping smoking (see section in this chapter on 'What can I do to help myself?') there are relatively simple topical measures that can relieve both systemic and discoid forms of lupus rash. Topical corticosteroids such as clobetasol and clobetasone are effective—although the higher strength forms should be used sparingly and for limited periods—and topical tacrolimus may also be used. Oral antimalarials (principally hydroxychloroquine, but chloroquine and mepacrine are also used) are also effective and are recommended in patients with a persistent rash. Severe cases with a widespread or refractory rash may need oral corticosteroids and/or immunosuppressants. In general, it is rarely necessary to use cyclophosphamide, mycophenolate, or biologics for skin lupus alone; although the skin may often be inflamed as part of a more general flare that is treated with such agents, and many patients with skin involvement were included in clinical trials of biologic agents.

Hair loss can be very difficult to reverse, especially if there is scarring alopecia, and some patients may need to wear wigs. It is important to consider whether there may be a separate cause for the alopecia (eg, iron deficiency, ageing, drug side effects). Oral hydroxychloroquine may also help.

Mouth ulcers in SLE are common and often painless and tolerated by patients without changes in medication. If severe enough to make eating difficult, oral corticosteroids are indicated.

Joint pain

Joint pain is very common in patients with SLE, but takes the form of arthralgia more commonly than overt inflammatory arthritis. It is important to remember that joint hypermobility and fibromyalgia, both much commoner conditions than SLE, may co-exist with lupus and can cause arthralgia and myalgia in these patients. There is a higher threshold for using disease modifying drugs such as methotrexate and sulfasalazine in SLE than in rheumatoid arthritis, because in SLE the joint pain is not usually associated with ongoing damage to bone and the development of deformities. Thus the use of medications in treating the musculoskeletal manifestations of SLE is primarily designed to control symptoms rather than to prevent damage. In many cases use of analgesics or non-steroidal anti-inflammatory drugs (NSAIDs), either regularly or on an 'as required' basis, is sufficient to provide this control. However, NSAIDs must be used with caution in patients with chronic renal insufficiency or with risk factors for cardiovascular disease. Antimalarials also have a beneficial effect on joint pain in patients with SLE. Corticosteroids, either oral or intramuscular, can be used to treat short-term flares of arthritis in patients with SLE (see section in this chapter on How can acute but limited flares of symptoms be managed?).

A minority of patients with SLE develop a pattern of persistent joint inflammation with morning stiffness, similar to that of rheumatoid arthritis. Some of these patients are also seropositive for rheumatoid factor or anti-cyclic citrullinated peptide antibodies and can be considered to have a true SLE/rheumatoid arthritis overlap syndrome. Where the arthritis is the dominant feature, these patients should be treated along the

Table 6.2 Management of mild SLE with intermittent flares	
Clinical problem	Management
Skin and hair involvement	Sun protection Topical corticosteroid Topical tacrolimus Antimalarials
Joint pain	Non-steroidal anti-inflammatory drugs (NSAIDs) Analgesics Antimalarials NB—watch out for SLE/rheumatoid arthritis over-lap, which may need to be treated as for rheumatoid arthritis with DMARDS/biologics
Chest pain due to pleurisy or pericarditis	Non-steroidal anti-inflammatory drugs
Flare of any of the above not responding to symptomatic treatment	Short course of oral corticosteroids (eg, 30 mg prednisolone daily reducing by 5 mg every 3–4 days to zero) or single dose of intramuscular depot corticosteroid (eg, methylprednisolone 80 mg or 120 mg)

same lines as patients with rheumatoid arthritis using disease modifying drugs, but the co-existence of SLE means that they may also need low-dose oral corticosteroids to control non-articular features. Anti-tumour necrosis factor agents are very rarely used in patients with SLE, but may sometimes be helpful in these overlap syndrome patients.

Fatigue

Fatigue is one of the most difficult symptoms to treat in SLE and may not respond to medications. This is because fatigue in these patients is often multi-factorial and not due solely to active inflammation caused by the disease. Anaemia of chronic disease, poor sleep, hypothyroidism (found in about 8% of patients with SLE) and fibromyalgia may all contribute. There is little definitive evidence that medications improve fatigue, though some patients experience improvement with either antimalarials or corticosteroids.

In summary, many patients with SLE live with a persistent low level of symptoms that do not represent inflammation threatening major organs and do not require treatment with high-dose corticosteroids or immunosuppressants. As summarized in Table 6.2, the mainstays of management in these patients are symptomatic and topical treatments and antimalarials.

How can acute but limited flares of symptoms be managed?

Many patients have persistent low-level symptoms (see section in this chapter, Management of mild SLE: What medications can help my everyday symptoms?), punc-tuated with flares of worse symptoms lasting a few days or weeks. Sometimes these flares may be precipitated by particular events, such as stressful episodes at home or work, infection, or exposure to ultra-violet radiation. Examples of such flares could include sudden worsening of rash, a polyarticular or monoarticular flare of joint inflam-mation, or an attack of chest pain and breathlessness due to pericarditis or pleurisy.

The aim of management during these flares is to bring them to an end quickly while using drugs sparingly. A single flare of this type should not lead to long-term corticosteroid and/or immunosuppressant treatment. The most effective agents to manage these flares are oral corticosteroids. A short course of oral prednisolone, starting at 20–30 mg per day and decreasing in steps of 5 mg every 3–4 days, such that the total course lasts for about a fortnight, is often effective. An alternative is to give a single intra-muscular dose of a depot preparation such as 80–120 mg methylprednisolone. Patients concerned about adverse effects of oral corticosteroids, such as weight gain, may particularly prefer this approach.

If flares of this kind are frequent enough that this type of treatment is being required 3–4 times a year or more, however, then the patient may be better served by taking regular oral prednisolone at a dose of 5 mg per day or below. If that dose is insufficient to prevent the flares then a combination of low dose prednisolone and azathioprine may be required.

What if my SLE becomes severe?

The implication of attending a specialist centre for regular follow-up and monitoring is that this will ensure early detection of episodes where the nature of the disease changes from a chronic mild condition to something more severe that can threaten the function of vital organs or even the patient's life. The most common scenario in which this happens is lupus nephritis, in which the standard of management is to use *both* corticosteroids and immunosuppressants, based on data from extensive clinical trials. Other forms of severe SLE, such as neuropsychiatric, gastrointestinal, and haematological involvement occur too rarely for large clinical trials to have been feasible. In these cases much of the evidence comes from retrospective case series and treatment is commonly with corticosteroids alone, immunosuppressants being reserved for refractory or particularly severe cases.

Renal SLE (lupus nephritis)

The clinical features and investigations in lupus nephritis are described in detail in Chapters 4 (Clinical features of SLE) and 5 (Laboratory tests and investigations). It suffices here to stress that many patients may have few or no symptoms at the time of diagnosis, presenting only with proteinuria, abnormal blood tests, and/or high blood pressure. It is important to be aware of this and not to under-treat patients or reduce the treatment too quickly on the grounds that the patient feels well. One should rather be guided by monitoring urine protein, serum albumin, and measures of disease activity (eg, erythrocyte sedimentation rate and level of anti-dsDNA antibodies). It is always advisable to carry out a renal biopsy where possible to establish the histological type of the nephritis and to show how much active inflammation, as opposed to chronic damage, is present in the glomeruli.

Thirty years ago, management of lupus nephritis was revolutionized by trials pioneered by the United States National Institutes of Health (NIH) showing that a combination of corticosteroid (oral or intravenous) and intravenous cyclophosphamide gave marked improvements in outcome. This led to development of the NIH regimen for lupus nephritis with oral corticosteroids accompanied by pulses of intravenous cyclophosphamide every month for six months, and then every three months for two years. Azathioprine, rather than cyclophosphamide was used for maintenance of remission. In long-term follow-up of 111 patients, the NIH regimen proved successful in reducing the rate of end-stage renal failure.[6] However, high dose cyclophosphamide is associated with problems of toxicity including cystitis, bone marrow suppression, and infertility so the NIH regimen is now rarely used. It has been replaced by either oral mycophenolate or the low-dose Euro-Lupus cyclophosphamide regimen.

There have been a number of trials comparing mycophenolate to cyclophosphamide in the management of SLE, most recently the Aspreva Lupus Management Study (ALMS) in which 370 patients with lupus nephritis were randomized to mycophenolate mofetil 3 g per day or intravenous cyclophosphamide (0.5 to 1 g/m^2) given in monthly pulses. Patients in both groups received oral corticosteroids tapering from a maximum starting dose of 60 mg prednisone per day. Over a 24-week follow-up period, both regimens were equally effective at reducing proteinuria and had equal risk of adverse effects.[7] A second paper describing non-renal outcomes in the same patients also showed that both forms of treatment were equally effective.[8]

The Euro-Lupus regimen involves six intravenous pulses of 500 mg cyclophosphamide at fortnightly intervals. A trial of 90 patients comparing this with the NIH regimen showed that both were equally effective in achieving renal remission and preventing renal flares.[9] In both arms of the study, azathioprine was given to maintain remission. Overall, either azathioprine or mycophenolate can be used in combination with low dose oral corticosteroids to maintain renal remission in lupus nephritis.[10] Azathioprine has advantages such as not being contraindicated in pregnancy. There is no definitive consensus regarding how long maintenance therapy should be continued and it is possible for flares of nephritis to occur even many years after the original presentation. Decisions about reducing or stopping therapy in patients in remission should be taken on a case-by-case basis taking into account factors such as activity of organs outside the kidney, urine protein level, the patient's desire for pregnancy, and adverse effects of drugs suffered by individual patients.

In summary: for proliferative lupus nephritis (Class III or IV), the best treatment options to induce remission are oral prednisolone starting at 30–40 mg/day and tapering over 6 months, together with either mycophenolate 2–3 g/day or the low dose cyclophosphamide regimen; and to maintain remission with low-dose oral prednisolone plus oral azathioprine or mycophenolate. Some lupus specialists prefer to give 2–3 pulses of intravenous methylprednisolone at the start of treatment followed by oral corticosteroids. Calcineurin inhibitors such as tacrolimus may be an effective alternative to mycophenolate or cyclophosphamide, especially in pure membranous lupus nephritis. In cases of lupus nephritis that do not respond to mycophenolate or the low-dose cyclophosphamide regimen, high-dose intravenous cyclophosphamide or rituximab should be considered.

International guidelines on management of lupus nephritis have been published both in the USA and Europe in the last few years. In this chapter, the European League Against Rheumatism (EULAR) guidelines have generally been followed.[11]

It is important to maintain good control of blood pressure in patients with previous lupus nephritis, as hypertension increases proteinuria. Ideally, the diastolic pressure should be kept below 80 mmHg using ACE inhibitors, angiotensin antagonists, calcium-channel inhibitors, or diuretics.

Severe non-renal SLE

Examples of severe non-renal SLE requiring urgent and aggressive treatment include neuropsychiatric SLE (eg, seizures, psychosis), lupus mesenteric vasculitis, severe haemolytic anaemia (Coombs positive with haemoglobin <8 g/dL), and thrombocytopenia (platelet count < 30 x 10^9/L). In all these situations, the mainstay of treatment

Table 6.3 Management of severe SLE	
Clinical problem	Management
Lupus nephritis	Induce remission with high-dose corticosteroids (oral/iv) plus either mycophenolate or low-dose cyclophosphamide regimen (500 mg iv, fortnightly x 6)
	Maintain remission with low dose corticosteroids (aim to reduce gradually to 5 mg per day) plus oral mycophenolate or oral azathioprine
	Consider tacrolimus instead of mycophenolate in Class V (membranous) lupus nephritis
	Consider rituximab in refractory cases
	Control blood pressure (aim for <80 mmHg diastolic)
Neuropsychiatric SLE	High-dose corticosteroids (iv or oral) will induce remission in most cases
	Refractory or severe cases may need iv cyclophosphamide
	Anticonvulsants or antipsychotics if required
Haematological SLE (especially anaemia or thrombocytopenia)	High-dose corticosteroids (iv or oral) will induce remission in most cases
	Refractory or severe cases may need iv cyclophosphamide or rituximab
	Transfusions of red cells or platelets if required
Lupus mesenteric vasculitis	High-dose intravenous steroids (patients usually have acute abdomen and are nil by mouth)
	Refractory or severe cases may need iv cyclophosphamide
	Surgery is rarely needed

is to use high-dose corticosteroids (either oral or intravenous) together with specific therapy for the particular organ involved. For example anticonvulsants or antipsychotics may be needed in neuropsychiatric SLE, and transfusions in haematological SLE. Most cases of lupus mesenteric vasculitis can be managed without surgery.[12] Splenectomy is almost never required for thrombocytopenia now that biologics such as rituximab are available.

In those cases that are either life-threatening at onset or where corticosteroids alone do not achieve remission, immunosuppression is added. Intravenous cyclophosphamide is a common choice and there are data supporting its use in both neuropsychiatric lupus,[13] and lupus mesenteric vasculitis.[12]

Patients who have recovered from severe non-renal lupus are often maintained on low-dose oral corticosteroids +/− azathioprine long-term to prevent relapses.

Management of severe renal and non-renal SLE is summarized in Table 6.3.

Will I get side effects from my lupus medications?

Many of the medications use to treat patients with SLE can have side effects and, given that these drugs are often taken for many years, the risk/benefit ratio for these drugs is an important consideration. Corticosteroids can cause a multitude of adverse effects including weight gain, hirsutism, cataracts, diabetes mellitus, and hypertension. Some of the more visible side effects may add to the distress experienced by patients with SLE about their appearance, whereas less visible effects such as osteoporosis and hypertension may cause complications over the long term. Best practice is to use the lowest dose of corticosteroids compatible with maintaining control of disease activity. The ability to reduce corticosteroid dose may be limited by repeated flares of symptoms such as arthritis or pleurisy, or by the need to prevent flares of serious manifestations such as lupus nephritis. The possibility of osteopenia/osteoporosis should be considered in all patients on long-term corticosteroids, especially those taking high doses and those who are post-menopausal women. Although some authors have suggested that vitamin D treatment could help reduce disease activity in SLE, the evidence for this is not convincing; however, vitamin D levels should be maintained (by giving supplements if necessary) in osteopenic patients. The introduction of biologics such as rituximab in early disease holds promise for allowing use of corticosteroids in lupus to be minimized or avoided.[14] This is discussed further in Chapter 7 (Biologic therapies in SLE).

There are arguments for treating all patients with SLE with hydroxychloroquine long-term, even if asymptomatic. These arguments come chiefly from observational studies showing that hydroxychloroquine treatment is associated with less development of damage in patients with SLE over time, as well as from a small Canadian randomized trial showing that withdrawal of hydroxychloroquine was associated with increased risk of lupus flare.[15] On the other hand, there is a very small risk of retinal toxicity associated with long-term use of hydroxychloroquine. There is no definite consensus on the issue and a fair compromise may be to continue this drug long term in all patients who have no side effects. There is no good evidence that retinal screening is beneficial in the first 5–7 years of taking hydroxychloroquine, but after that it is reasonable to suggest annual retinal screening by an optician or ophthalmologist.

Patients taking mycophenolate, azathioprine, or cyclophosphamide require monitoring of full blood count. Plans for pregnancy should be discussed with all patients who are being started on mycophenolate or cyclophosphamide. Mycophenolate is contraindicated in pregnancy and cyclophosphamide may cause reduced fertility. These issues are discussed further in Chapter 9 (Management of special situations in SLE).

What if I have antiphospholipid syndrome as well as SLE?

Between 30–40% of patients with lupus have antiphospholipid antibodies in their serum. Some, but not all of these patients develop antiphospholipid syndrome (APS) in addition to SLE. Between 10–15% of patients with SLE have APS. The features of APS are vascular thrombosis, which may be arterial or venous, and pregnancy loss. Patients may suffer recurrent miscarriages. APS may also occur separately from SLE (primary APS). The only evidence-based treatment for preventing recurrent vascular thrombosis in APS is long-term anticoagulation.[16] The intensity of anticoagulation depends on whether the thromboses are venous or arterial. Pregnant women with APS are managed with aspirin and daily subcutaneous heparin injections. In managing a patient who has both SLE and APS, it is important to be clear that both conditions are managed separately. Immunosuppressants and corticosteroids given for SLE do not reduce the risk of thrombosis in APS, and anticoagulation has no effect on SLE disease activity. Thus, a patient with SLE and APS should be treated with the appropriate intensity of anticoagulation whether their lupus is quiescent, mild, or severe.

References

1. Rees F, Doherty M, Grainge M, Davenport G, Lanyon P, Zhang W. The incidence and prevalence of systemic lupus erythematosus in the UK, 1999–2012. *Ann Rheum Dis*. doi: 10.1136/annrheumdis-2014-206334. Epub 29 Sep 2014.

2. Abu-Shakra M, Urowitz MB, Gladman DD, Gough J. Mortality studies in systemic lupus ery-thematosus. Results from a single center. II. Predictor variables for mortality. *J Rheumatol* 1995;22:1265–70.

3. Hochberg MC. Updating the American College of Rheumatology revised criteria for the clas-sification of systemic lupus erythematosus. *Arthritis Rheum* 1997;40:1725.

4. Elliott JR, Manzi S, Edmundowicz D. The role of preventive cardiology in systemic lupus ery-thematosus. *Curr Rheumatol Rep* 2007;9:125–30.

5. Tench CM, McCarthy J, McCurdie I, White PD, D'Cruz DP. Fatigue in systemic lupus erythe-matosus: a randomized controlled trial of exercise. *Rheumatology* (Oxford). 2003;42:1050–4.

6. Steinberg AD, Steinberg SC. Long-term preservation of renal function in patients with lupus nephritis receiving treatment that includes cyclophosphamide versus those treated with pred-nisone only. *Arthritis Rheum.* 1991;34:945–50.

7. Isenberg D, Appel GB, Contreras G, et al. Influence of race/ethnicity on response to lupus nephritis treatment: the ALMS study. *Rheumatology* (Oxford). 2010;49:128–40.

8. Ginzler EM, Wofsy D, Isenberg D, et al. Nonrenal disease activity following mycophenolate mofetil or intravenous cyclophosphamide as induction treatment for lupus nephritis: findings in a multicenter, prospective, randomized, open-label, parallel-group clinical trial. *Arthritis Rheum* 2010;62:211–21.

9. Houssiau FA, Vasconcelos C, D'Cruz D, et al. Immunosuppressive therapy in lupus nephri-tis: the Euro-Lupus Nephritis Trial, a randomized trial of low-dose versus high-dose intrave-nous cyclophosphamide. *Arthritis Rheum* 2002;46:2121–31.

10. Contreras G, Pardo V, Leclercq B, 'et al. Sequential therapies for proliferative lupus nephritis. *N Engl J Med* 2004;350:971–80.

11. Bertsias GK, Tektonidou M, Amoura Z, et al. Joint European League Against Rheumatism and European Renal Association-European Dialysis and Transplant Association (EULAR/ ERA-EDTA) recommendations for the management of adult and paediatric lupus nephritis. *Ann Rheum Dis* 2012;71:1771–82.

12. Yuan S, Ye Y, Chen D, et al. Lupus mesenteric vasculitis: clinical features and associated factors for the recurrence and prognosis of disease. *Semin Arthritis Rheum* 2014;43:759–66.

13. Neuwelt CM, Lacks S, Kaye BR, Ellman JB, Borenstein DG. Role of intravenous cyclophos-phamide in the treatment of severe neuropsychiatric systemic lupus erythematosus. *Am J Med* 1995;98:32–41.

14. Condon MB, Ashby D, Pepper RJ, et al. Prospective observational single-centre cohort study to evaluate the effectiveness of treating lupus nephritis with rituximab and mycophenolate mofetil but no oral steroids. *Ann Rheum Dis* 2013;72:1280–6.

15. CanadianHydroxychloroquineStudyGroup. A randomized study of the effect of with-drawing hydroxychloroquine sulfate in systemic lupus erythematosus. The Canadian Hydroxychloroquine Study Group. *N Engl J Med* 1991;324:150–4.

16. Lim W, Crowther MA, Eikelboom JW. Management of antiphospholipid antibody syn-drome: a systematic review. *JAMA* 2006;295:1050–7.

Chapter 7

Biologic therapies in systemic lupus erythematosus

Maria Mouyis and David Isenberg

Key points

- SLE is a multi-systemic autoimmune disease requiring aggressive treatment. Traditional treatments have improved the prognosis in SLE but are limited by side effects and patient tolerability.
- Understanding the pathogenesis of SLE has led to a new treatment era of biologic therapies.
- Current biologic therapies target B cells, anti-B cell activating factors, T cell activation, and anti-interferon alpha.
- Treatment with biologic therapies is associated with an increased infection rate, possible reactivation of tuberculosis, and immunosuppression.
- Rituximab is one of the first biologics to be used in the treatment of SLE.

Introduction

As detailed in the earlier chapters, systemic lupus erythematosus (SLE) has multiple manifestations ranging from mild disease requiring little treatment, to severe clinical disease requiring admission to an intensive care unit. An increased understanding in the pathogenesis of the disease has allowed the development of treatment options from conventional disease-modifying immunosuppressive drugs to biologic agents that target particular cells or molecules. An ideal SLE drug would have a good safety profile and improve disease control. This improvement is best 'captured' by objective disease activity scores.

Traditionally the objective of SLE therapy is to minimize disease activity. In the 1950s clinicians used aspirin, chloroquine, and corticosteroids to treat SLE. In the 1960s azathioprine and methotrexate became more widely available. At the National Institute of Health in the United States, regimes incorporating cyclophosphamide came to the fore in the 1970s to treat lupus nephritis. With some exceptions (eg, mycophenolate) few new conventional drugs have been introduced in the past 25 years. Management depends on the clinical manifestations of SLE. As described in Chapter 6 (Conventional treatments in SLE), well-established therapies for different clinical manifestations of the disease range from hydroxychloroquine and low dose oral prednisone, to methotrexate, azathioprine, cyclophosphamide, and mycophenolate mofetil in response to different clinical disease manifestations.[1] These traditional disease-modifying, anti-rheumatic drugs (DMARDs) have significantly improved patient survival in SLE but, as mentioned, have significant side effects which can be life threatening and not all patients respond adequately. The development of targeted biologic therapy has opened the prospects for a new era in SLE therapy.

To date, few clinical trials have effectively compared conventional therapies. The more successful management of clinical disease in the past 40 years has been made possible by the use of dialysis and in some cases organ transplantation, principally renal transplantation. Controlling the complications of SLE (such as osteoporosis, hypotension, and cardiovascular disease) has dramatically improved the clinical course of the disease. The biologic therapies used to date, principally rituximab and belimumab, have proved useful in refractory SLE, but do themselves have side effects (see 'safety profile' subsection in this chapter for rituximab and belimumab). The biggest concern for both conventionally treated patients and those given biologics remains that of infection, owing to their immunosuppressant effects.

Advantages and disadvantages of biologics in SLE

Evidence from long-term studies suggests that we have reached the best outcome we are likely to obtain with conventional drugs and supportive therapies.[2] The potential advantage of biologic therapy is its potential effectiveness in terms of disease control. They also do not have to be stopped in the pre-pregnancy phase unlike methotrexate, cyclophosphamide, and mycophenolate mofetil, but the evidence regarding the safety of these drugs during pregnancy is inconclusive. Disadvantages include: allergic or transfusion reaction; infection, including mycobacterium tuberculosis (which usually occurs within the first 6 months); and hepatitis B and C reactivation. A very rare but significant risk of rituximab is the development of JC (John Cunningham) virus infection which causes progressive, multifocal, leucoencephalopathy (PML) but virtually all immunosuppressive drugs have been linked to PML—the implication being that it is not a drug-specific effect.[3] An ongoing problem is the formation of antibodies to the biologics, especially those that are not fully humanized. Variable rates exist between the different agents and they are not all functionally significant. The incidence of this phenomenon is reduced with the concomitant use of methotrexate.

A key challenge to the introduction of biologic therapy to treat patients with SLE is the cost. Most of these agents are not formally approved globally and in the UK the National Institute for Health and Care Excellence (NICE) exists to determine not so much whether a drug is effective but rather if it is cost effective.

Pathogenesis

To understand how biologic agents work, one must understand the pathogenesis of SLE (see Figure 7.1 (see colour version on inside cover)).[4] SLE is multifactorial in its origins. Genetic, hormonal, and environmental components almost certainly interact in a variety of ways to induce the broad diversity of clinical manifestations. Chapter 2 (Aetiopathogenesis of SLE) provides a detailed account of these components.

Briefly, B lymphocyte abnormalities are clearly a major driver of the events that lead to lupus. A variety of other cells and abnormalities involved in efficient apoptosis, also play a major role. This diversity of cells and processes presents a number of therapeutic opportunities, facilitated by the technology that has driven the 'biologics revolution'. Figure 7.1 provides an indication of those cells and molecules which are targeted by biologic agents.

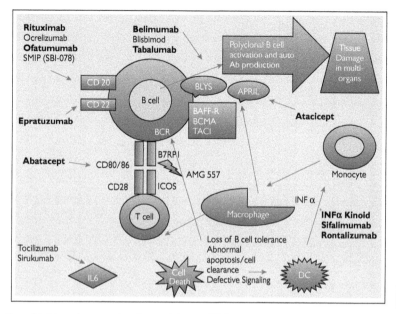

Figure 7.1 Schematic presentation of targeted therapy of SLE.

Modified from Recent developments in the treatment of patients with systemic lupus erythematosus: focusing on biologic therapies, Zozik Fattah and David A Isenberg, Expert opinion on biological therapy (2014) Vol. 14, No. 3, 311–326, reprinted with permission of Taylor and Francis.

(See colour version on inside cover.)

Biologic therapies

As indicated in Figure 7.1 there are several biologics which act on B cells. These various biologic agents are discussed in detail below. Table 7.1 summarizes the doses used, mechanism of action, and side effect profile of each biologic agent. Each biologic is prescribed with premedication including corticosteroids, antihistamines, and paracetamol to minimize infusion-related and allergic type reactions.

Biologic therapies affecting B cells

Anti-CD20: rituximab and Ofatumumab

Anti-CD22: epratuzumab

Rituximab

Mechanism of action Rituximab is a chimeric/humanized monoclonal antibody that acts on CD20+ cells and leads to B cell depletion. The CD20 antigen is found on surface of pre-B cells which mature to memory B cells, at which point (before they develop into plasma cells) the marker is lost. The mechanism of action is via apoptosis and complement activation. The response to rituximab is reliant on a decline in the number of B cells and how quickly auto-reactive plasma cells develop. Paradoxically, rituximab may be associated with an increase in the B-lymphocyte stimulating factor (also known as B cell activating factor, BAFF) in some patients which increases the reconstitution of B cells.[5–7]

Table 7.1 An overview of biologic therapy in SLE

Biologic agent	Mechanism of action	Dose	Side effects	Approval	Trial	Comments
Rituximab	Anti CD20 chimeric monoclonal antibody	1 g × 2: 2 weeks apart 375 mg/m² every 4 weeks 750 mg cyclophosphamide may be given with the first infusion to increase B cell depletion effect.	Infusion reaction Increased infection risk PML Lymphoma	NHS England	EXPLORER LUNAR	Problems with trial design and use of immunosuppressives and glucocorticoids
Belimumab	Human monoclonal immunoglobulin (IgG1γ)	10 mg/kg every 2 weeks × 3, and then once every 4 weeks	Nausea Diarrhoea Headaches URTI Fever Cystitis Infusion reaction	NHS England FDA (USA) 2011	BLISS 52 BLISS 76	Prolonged onset of action, Not approved in renal and cerebral SLE. No BILAG scores.
Ofatumumab	Fully human monoclonal antibody against membrane proximal epitope on CD20 molecule	300 mg, 700 mg, 1000 mg over 24 weeks. With 2 weeks between each dose.	Infusion reactions Urticaria Rash Rhinitis Nausea URTI Headaches Fatigue Flushing	IFR	RA trials. Case reports in SLE	Used RA and chronic lymphocytic leukaemia
Epratuzumab	Monoclonal antibody, IgG1 against CD22 molecule	360 mg/m² every 2 weeks × 4 cycles	Infusion reaction Nausea Fatigue Generalized aches	IFR	EMBLEM Embody ALLEVIATE	Immunomodulatory

Sifalimumab	Anti-interferon (IFN)-alpha monoclonal antibody.	0.3, 1.0, 3.0, or 10.0 mg/kg—still undergoing trials.	Infusion reaction Fatigue URTI UTI Sinusitis Dizziness Arthralgia Headache Lymphopenia Anaemia	Phase III trial	Phase III trial	No data available in severe SLE
Atacicept	TACI-Ig fusion protein that inhibits BLyS and APRIL	150 mg weekly	LRTI/URTI Injection site reaction Fever Arthralgia Sinusitis Headache Fatigue Rhinitis Dizziness Depression	Phase III trial for non renal lupus August 1 and 2	Phase III trial	Infections and lower immunoglobulin levels in patient receiving concomitant mycophenolate mofetil.
Rontalizumab	A recombinant humanized monoclonal antibody to IFN-α	750 mg IV 4 weekly 300 mg SCT 2 weekly 0.3–10 mg/kg	Viral infections Reactivation herpes Sinusitis Bronchitis	Phase II trial	Phase II trial	
Abatacept	Human IgG1 heavy chain fused with CTLA4 that blocks T cell activation by B cells.	10–30 mg/kg	Nausea Headache Infusion reaction Fever Hypertension Back pain Infections	IFR	Phase III trials	Approved for the use of rheumatoid arthritis

Abbreviations: FDA: Federal Drug Administration, USA; IFR: individual funding request form; IV: intravenous; LRTI: lower respiratory tract infection; PML: progressive multifocal leucoencephalopathy; RA: rheumatoid arthritis; SCT: subcutaneous; URTI: upper respiratory tract infection; UTI: urinary tract infection.

Efficacy Numerous case reports and case series have reported significant clinical improvements in almost two thirds of patients given rituximab. However, two large-scale international trials, EXPLORER (studying non-renal patients)[8] and LUNAR (investigating patients with nephritis)[9] have proved disappointing because the primary end points were not met. There are various possibilities to explain this failure, but it is likely to be related to the concomitant use of large doses of glucocorticoids and immunosuppressants. Rituximab is widely used for the treatment of most forms of SLE, and has been used since 2000 in an off-licence capacity for refractory disease. The off-licence use of rituximab was assessed in a meta-analysis between 2002 and 2007. Nine studies and 26 case reports indicated that 188 patients were treated with rituximab for active SLE. Different therapeutic regimes were used including 375 mg/m^2 of rituximab, weekly for 4 weeks (39%); or two 1000-mg doses, 2 weeks apart (19%). Induction therapy included the co-administration of intravenous (IV) methylprednisolone in 58 patients (31%) and intravenous cyclophosphamide (750 mg administered with the first and fourth doses of rituximab in 97 patients (52%). All three agents: rituximab, cyclophosphamide, and IV methylprednisolone were given to 41 patients (22%). The analysis of this data has led to the use of current dose regimens. 91% of patients were recorded as having a clinical response, that is, resolution of symptoms. Unfortunately due to the lack of standardization across studies no objective measures were identified, although it was noted that in all patients who received cyclophosphamide and rituximab there was a higher clinical response ($p < 0.001$).[10] The most objective clinical study was performed by Leandro et al.[11] Twenty-four patients who had refractory SLE were divided into two groups. Six patients were treated with 500 mg of rituximab 2 weeks apart and 18 patients were treated with 1000 mg, 2 weeks apart. Each patient received 750 mg cyclophosphamide and high dose oral corticosteroids for 2 weeks. The global British Isles Lupus Assessment Group (BILAG) score ($p < 0.001$), serum C3 ($p < 0.001$) and anti-dsDNA antibodies ($p < 0.002$) improved significantly 6 months after rituximab administration. Improvements in BILAG scores by 24% occurred within the first 6 months. Long-term follow-up of the 188 treated patients, found that 46 relapsed at a mean of 12 months after rituximab administration. The rate of relapse may be related to disease severity and return of B cell immunity. Twenty-four of the 46 patients were re-treated with rituximab. An 80% response rate was observed, thus suggesting the role of rituximab as a maintenance therapy. Overall, the off-label studies have indicated a high response rate of 90% and led to the development of randomized control studies (RCTs) which are discussed in the efficacy sections for each drug later in this chapter.

In the UK, NHS England has sanctioned the use of rituximab on an individual basis in patients who have failed two immunosuppressive agents and require intermittent high dose glucocorticoids. The European League against Rheumatism (EULAR) and The American College of Rheumatology (ACR) guidelines also recommend the use of rituximab in patients with active SLE nephritis resistant to conventional therapies.

An important clinical advantage of using rituximab is its steroid-sparing effect. The first study illustrating a steroid-sparing effect was published in 2011. Eight female patients with newly diagnosed SLE were treated with 1 g of rituximab, 2 weeks apart, with 125 mg of methylprednisolone and 1 dose of cylcophosphamide followed by maintenance azathioprine. Response to treatment was assessed using the BILAG disease activity index, serum anti-dsDNA antibody levels, C3, ESR, CD19 and a protein:creatinine ratio (PCR). These parameters were tested at 0, 1, 3, 6, and 12 months. Results were compared with three SLE patients, matched for ethnicity, age, sex, disease onset, and disease duration who were treated with conventional therapy. At 6 months the group who received rituximab had a lower cumulative dose of prednisolone (1278.3 mg) compared with the control group (2834.6 mg), highlighting that early treatment with B cell depletion therapy can reduce the overall steroid burden.[12] This was further explored by Condon et al. who treated a cohort of 50 patients with lupus nephritis (biopsy proven class III, IV, or V) with 1 g of rituximab, 2 weeks apart, and 500 mg of intravenous methylprednisolone.[13] No oral steroids were given and mycophenolate mofetil was used as maintenance therapy. Remission was defined as a serum creatinine level of no greater than 15% above baseline and a urine PCR <50 mg/mmol. 70% ($n = 36$) of the patients achieved remission in a mean time of 36 weeks and only 2/50 patients required them in a 2-year follow-up period. Eleven patients flared at the median time of 65 weeks from remission. This study suggests that oral steroids can be avoided and B cell depletion might be considered early in the treatment of lupus nephritis and other systemic manifestations of SLE. However, confirmation of this open study is awaited. A current international trial comparing rituximab and mycophenolate with steroids and mycophenolate (the RITUXILIP study) should provide more definitive answers.

Safety profile Side-effects of rituximab include an infusion reaction which settles on stopping the infusion. Symptoms include fever, bronchospasm, rash, and hypotension. Post-rituximab monitoring is required to monitor for the development of infections such as tuberculosis (TB) and hepatitis B or C. The effect of B cell depletion lasts for 6–12 months in most cases. Accumulated doses may also cause hypogammaglobulinaemia, which may be linked to an increased risk of infection. Extremely rarely, progressive multifocal lymphadenopathy has developed in patients with SLE. However, it has also been reported following conventional immunosuppressive therapy and is not increased post rituximab. Post-B cell depletion, it is recommended that immunoglobulin and $CD19^+$ B cell counts are checked every 2 months until the B cell count has returned to normal.[7]

Ofatumamab

Mechanism of action Ofatumumab is a fully humanized monoclonal antibody against $CD20^+$ B cells and leads to B cell depletion. Unlike rituximab, however, there is greater complement dependant cytotoxicity.[7]

Efficacy It is used in the treatment of chronic lymphocytic leukaemia (CLL). In the United States it is used off-label for the treatment of patients with rheumatoid arthritis whose treatment with methotrexate has failed. Most studies assessing efficacy have been done in patients with rheumatoid arthritis although there are individual case reports indicating disease efficacy in SLE.[14]

Safety profile The main side effect is considered to be infusion-related reactions such as flushing, nausea, rhinitis, pruritus, upper respiratory tract infection, hypertension, and urticaria. The use of premedication with antihistamine and steroids may decrease the incidence of infusion-related reactions.[7] No case of PML has been reported to date.

Epratuzumab

Mechanism of action CD22 is a B cell transmembrane glycoprotein that is found on mature B cells, but not on memory or plasma cells. It is involved in B cell regulation and activation. Epratuzumab is an IgG1 monoclonal antibody that targets the CD22 molecule. This generates a positive signal that induces the natural inhibitory effect of

CD22 signalling on B cell activation. There is an estimated 40% reduction in the peripheral B cell count in patients with SLE post epratuzumab treatment.[7,15]

Efficacy It has more of an immunomodulatory effect compared with other biologic agents. Similar to rituximab it has a corticosteroid-sparing side effect as seen in the ALLEVIATE study. At week 24, mean cumulative corticosteroid doses with epratuzumab 360 and 720 mg/m² were at least 100 mg less than placebo.[16] It has been tested not only in patients with SLE, but also Sjogren's syndrome. A total of 227 patients in the EMBLEM study (a phase II trial),[17] with moderate/severe lupus on standard of care treatment were divided into six treatment groups: placebo or epratuzumab given as: 100 mg on alternate weeks; 400 mg on alternate weeks; 600 mg weekly; 1200 mg on alternate weeks; or 1800 mg on alternate weeks. The most effective dose over a 12-week period was found to be 600 mg weekly (a cumulative dose of 2400 mg) as evidenced by a BILAG-based composite lupus assessment (BICLA) at week 12, with 45.9% responders versus 21.1% responders on placebo ($p = 0.03$). A dosing regimen of 1200 mg on alternate weeks (also a 2400 mg cumulative dose) resulted in a slightly lower proportion of responders (40.5%; $p = 0.07$) but the study was powered to compare groups. Studies to date have not shown a significant decrease in autoantibody levels, only a partial reduction in B cells and no decrease in immunoglobulins; although disease activity did improve.

Very sadly, in July 2015 UCB-Pharma announced that their two, large-scale, phase III clinical trials assessing the efficacy of epratuzumab in patients with severe SLE (Embody 1 and 2) (NCT01261793; www.clinicaltrials.gov) failed to meet their primary end points. Full disclosure of the trial data will be published in due course. This casts the future of the drug into doubt.

Safety profile The side effect profile has been described from phase II trials and includes infusion reactions, fatigue, nausea, and non-specific pain in SLE patients. Patients with Sjogren's syndrome may experience swelling of the nasal mucosa and increased pressure in the glottis. Compared with placebo groups, there was no increased incidence of side effects.[15,17]

Anti-B cell activating factors

Belimumab

Mechanism of action B-lymphocyte stimulator (BLyS) is a transmembrane protein and part of the tumour necrosis factor (TNF) family. BlyS (also known as BAFF, B cell activating factor) is expressed by T cells, dendritic cells, and neutrophils. It binds to three receptors on the B cell surface: the B cell maturation antigen (BMCA), BR3, and a transmembrane activator and calcium modulating ligand interactor (TACI). Its function is to promote B cell maturation via these receptors. Over-expression of BLyS is seen in patients with SLE leading to an increased production of B cells and autoantibodies. Belimumab, fully humanized monoclonal antibody, is a B-lymphocyte stimulator inhibitor (BLyS) which prevents the maturation of B cells into plasma cells and subsequent production of antibodies.[15]

Efficacy BLISS 76 and BLISS 52 were the trials that showed belimumab to be effective in reducing flares and disease activity.[18,19] It was found to be most effective in patients with musculoskeletal and cutaneous involvement, associated with positive anti-nuclear antibodies/double-stranded DNA antibodies (ANA/dsDNA) and a low C3. Although belimumab was approved in 2011 by the US Food and Drug Administration for mild SLE, it is not approved for the treatment of active lupus nephritis or cerebral lupus (patients with lupus nephritis and cerebral lupus were excluded from the trials). It can be used in patients with active skin and joint SLE despite treatment with conventional therapies. The disadvantage of belimumab is its prolonged onset of action, therefore not an ideal agent for treatment of an acute flare. Corticosteroids would still be the treatment of choice in an acute flare. It takes approximately 6 months to achieve 70% of B cell depletion. The efficacy also depends on the levels of circulating BLyS/BAFF which vary between patients.

BLISS 52 was an international study lasting 52 weeks including Central and Eastern Europe, Asia-Pacific, and Latin America. At 52 weeks, 51% had a positive clinical response when treated with belilumab 1 mg/kg ($p = 0.01$), whereas the 10 mg/kg dose regimen resulted in 58% of responders ($p < 0.01$), compared with 44% responders in those given placebo (all patients received standard therapy as well).[18]

BLISS 76 was a 76-week study based in North America, and Western and Central Europe. At 52 weeks, 41%, 43%, and 34% of those treated with 1 mg/kg, 10 mg/kg, and placebo met the response respectively. In this study the results with the 1mg/kg dose did not reach statistical significance but at 10 mg/kg a p-value of 0.02 was noted. This response was not maintained at 76 weeks however, and at this time-point there was no statistically significant difference between the different groups. Post hoc analyses suggested that the patients most likely to benefit were those with high dsDNA antibody levels and a low C3 level at baseline.

Further analysis of the data suggested that belimumab may be less effective in patients of black ethnicity.[15] After seven years of open-label treatment (in a relatively small number of patients) the advantages for using belimumab in SLE include: a) an improvement in active disease; b) a decrease in anti-dsDNA antibody titres of 70% from baseline; c) a steroid-sparing effect; and d) a low rate of adverse events. However, the suggestion that serologically active patients would do better was not confirmed and the high cost of the drug (approximately $30,000 per year in the USA) is a major obstacle to its widespread acceptance.[20] Trials assessing its effectiveness in renal disease and in black patients are ongoing.

Safety profile A meta-analysis showed a well-tolerated safety profile. Reported side effects include nausea, diarrhoea, upper respiratory tract infections, headaches, viral gastroenteritis, cystitis, and infusion reactions. The risk of infection is thought to be related to changes in signalling pathways as low BLyS levels lead to a reduction in TACI signalling which reduces host defence against encapsulated bacteria. The severity of infection was not dose-related and was similar to placebo. Although deemed safe there is one report of fatal anaphylaxis in 2012, hence there is a risk of delayed acute hypersensitivity reaction.[18,20]

Tabalumab

Mechanism of action Tabalumab is a human IgG4 monoclonal antibody. It targets both membrane-bound and soluble BAFF.[15]

Efficacy and safety profile Tabalumab is designed to provide an alternative option that acts against membrane-bound and soluble BAFF, whereas belimumab acts against membrane-bound BAFF only. Tabalumab may also be given as a subcutaneous injection as opposed to an intravenous infusion such as belimumab. The loading dose of tabalumab is 240 mg, followed by 120 mg every 2 weeks or 4 weeks in combination with traditional SLE treatments. (NIHR HSC ID: 5581)

Phase III trials called IILUMINATE I and 2 undertaken by Eli Lilly were recently completed. The primary end point assessing SLE disease activity and response (SLE responder index 5) was met in the second study, but overall the collective data were not considered by the company to be significantly impressive to support further work with the drug. The release of the trial data is currently pending (Tabalumab in Systemic Lupus Erythematosus; NIHR HSC ID: 5581 at http://www.evidence.nhs.uk).

Atacicept

Mechanism of action Atacicept is a TACI-Ig fusion receptor protein that inhibits BLyS and a proliferation-inducing ligand (APRIL), thereby reducing B cell proliferation, interferon gamma, and immunoglobulin production. It is a novel agent as it affects both BLyS and APRIL simultaneously. By blocking both cytokines memory cells are spared, but there is a decreased survival of mature B cells and plasma cells.[15]

Efficacy In a phase Ib double blinded study, atacicept was given to 47 patients with mild to moderate SLE. A dose-response reduction in B lymphocytes was noticed after a transient increase, and immunoglobulin levels were reduced, but more noticeably the IgM levels were reduced.[21] A subsequent phase II/III trial to assess the reduction of flares was performed.[22] Patients with active disease achieved remission (no BILAG As or Bs) using corticosteroids. They were then given a higher (150 mg) or lower (75 mg) dose of atacicept or placebo. Towards the end of the trial the higher dose arm was, probably erroneously, prematurely terminated due to two fatal pulmonary infections. Both doses of atacicept demonstrated significant improvement in the C3 and anti-dsDNA antibody levels. Furthermore, post hoc analysis showed that patients receiving 150 mg, as opposed to 75 mg or placebo, had a significant (43%) reduction of flares, $p = 0.027$. There was also a delayed time to flare ($p = 0.009$) in those given the higher dose.

Safety profile The side effect profile is listed in Table 7.1. Side effects do not appear to be dose dependant. Overall the percentage of deaths in this trial was identical to that seen in the belimumab trials. In an earlier trial using atacicept and mycophenolate mofetil there appeared to be an increase in infections but this was related to the hypogammaglobulinaemia caused by mycophenolate mofetil.[4] Trials in rheumatoid arthritis using atacicept were not associated with deaths due to significant infections. Infections include *Haemophilus influenza* pneumonia, *Legionella* pneumonia, and *Bacillus* bacteraemia. Preclinical studies showed an increase in liver transaminases.

Comparing different biological studies, the infection rates were almost identical in BLISS 76 (7.35%) compared with atacicept 150 mg arm (6.9%).[23] The use of rituximab in the EXPLORER trial had an infection rate of 9.5%.[24]

Anti-interferon alpha

Interferons form part of the large cytokine family. The various types of interferons will act on interferon receptors I, II, and III. Interferons can modulate the function of the immune system depending on which receptor they bind to. Stimulation of the Interferon I receptor promotes signalling of TNFα and an increase in B cell activating factors (BAFF). It is important to note that this is not an SLE-specific phenomenon but a function of the immune system.

Studies of pathogenesis suggest that in SLE there are higher levels of interferon (IFN)-regulated gene expression, which in turn promotes high levels of BAFF, B cell maturation, antibody production, T cell activation and, as a result, inflammation. The development of IFNα monoclonal antibodies allows for the blockade of type I IFN receptors through the neutralization of IFNα subtypes. Reductions in gene expression will down-regulate the inflammatory cytokine pathways. Type I IFN inducible genes in SLE patients have been used as biomarkers to assess treatment response. Recovery of gene expression occurs approximately 6 months after the last dose.[7,15]

Sifalimumab

Mechanism of action Sifalimumab is an anti-IFNα monoclonal antibody. This drug is currently in phase III trials. The results to date report that Sifalimumab serum levels increase in a dose-dependent manner, which in turn leads to a dose-dependent inhibition of type 1 IFN gene expression.

Efficacy A phase IIb, randomized, double blind, placebo-controlled study in patients with active SLE met its primary end points.[25] Four hundred and thirty-one patients were randomized to receiving monthly Sifalimumab in doses of 200 mg, 600 mg, or 1200 mg, or placebo for a 1-year period. The primary end point was to show a reduction in SLE activity using the SLE responder index. There were 58.3%, 65.5%, and 59.8% responders found in the 200 mg, 600 mg, 1200 mg groups respectively, versus 45% responders in the placebo group (a *p*-value of 0.031 was demonstrated when comparing 1200 mg versus placebo). Phase III trials are currently underway.

Safety profile Side effects include infusion reactions, nausea, upper respiratory tract infections, urinary tract infections, headache, arthralgia, and reported cases of herpes zoster. It is generally considered to have a good safety profile.[7,25]

Rontalizumab

Mechanism of action Rontalizumab is a recombinant humanized monoclonal antibody.

Efficacy Patients with moderate to severe non renal lupus were assessed in a randomized, double blind, placebo-controlled study. The efficacy and safety of rontalizumab (ROSE) study was first presented at the ACR, but the extended report was recently published.[26] On entry into the study, patients had a moderate to severe flare. All immunosuppressive agents except corticosteroids and hydroxychloroquine were stopped. Patients were given 750 mg intravenously, 300 mg subcutaneously, or a placebo over a period of 2–4 weeks. There was no difference in disease activity assessed on the BILAG index 2004 (primary end point), and the SLE response index (SRI; secondary end point) at 24 weeks, but there was a lower steroid burden and fewer flares in the rontalizumab group of patients with low levels of interferon signature metric (gene expression). A decrease in the expression of interferon (IFN)-regulated genes (IRGs) was noted, but not in the level of dsDNA or levels of IFN-inducible proteins. Levels of interferon signature increased as the drug levels decreased.[15,26]

Safety profile This drug demonstrates an acceptable safety profile in the early stages of use. One case of leukaemia was reported in the study as well an increase in viral infections (See Table 7.1).[25]

Blockade of T cell activation

Abatacept

Mechanism of action Abatacept (Orencia) is a fusion protein. Human IgG1 is fused to CTLA4 which is a T-cell surface receptor. The CTLA4 binds to the B cell, thus preventing T cell membrane CTLA4A and CD28 from binding to the receptor. This prevents B cell activation and T cell-mediated cytokine release.[7,15]

Efficacy In murine studies of lupus nephritis, treatment with a combination of abatacept and cyclophosphamide improved mortality, and reduced antibody titres and proteinuria. Human trials in SLE have been less successful.[15] A phase II/III trial assessing abatcept in lupus nephritis did not meet the primary end points of inactive urinary sediment, minimal proteinuria, and maintenance of glomerular filtration rate over 52 weeks (ie, complete remission). Abatacept (10 mg/kg or 30 mg/kg) was added to mycophenolate mofetil and high dose steroids. Although the primary outcome was not met, treatment with abatacept resulted in a 20–30% reduction of proteinuria as well as improvements in anti-dsDNA antibody and complement levels.[27] Wolfsy et al. applied the LUNAR trial response criteria to the same data and found a 20% response rate in the abatacept arm compared with placebo (6%)[28] emphasizing the need for those designing clinical trials to set realistic end points (as well as minimizing the concomitant steroids and immunosuppressants).

Safety profile As with other biologics, infections are a cause for concern. Associated side effects include nausea, headache, infusion reaction, fever, hypertension, back pain, and infections.[7] There was no significant increase of side effects compared with the placebo group. 96% of reactions are thought to be mild or moderate and related to infection.

Future possibilities

Anti-complement therapies: Eculizumab

This is a fully humanized IgG2/IgG4 monoclonal antibody that has undergone phase 1 trials in SLE. It is directed against C5, inhibiting C5 to C5a and C5b, thereby preventing the formation of the terminal membrane attack complex. This effect in turn reduces complement-mediated injury to glomerular cells. It has been shown to reduce proteinuria and improve renal histology in lupus nephritis. Further trials are required to assess the potential efficacy of this treatment.[15,29]

Conclusion

The use of precisely targeted biologic drugs offers hope for those lupus patients who have failed to respond to conventional treatment. However, several failed trials mean that the role of biologic therapy still needs to be further defined. The objective of SLE treatment is to induce remission, prevent end organ damage, and maintain cost effectiveness. New biologic therapies are likely to change the management of SLE in years to come with or without conventional DMARDs. As our understanding of the pathogenesis continues to increase so new agents will be developed.

References

1. Bertsias G, Ioannidis JPA, Boletis J, et al. EULAR recommendations for the management of systemic lupus erythematosus. Report of a task force of the EULAR standing committee for international clinical studies including therapeutics. *Ann Rheum Dis* 2008;67:195–205.

2. Croca SC, Rodrigues T, Isenberg DA. Assessment of a lupus nephritis cohort over a 30-year period. *Rheumatology* (Oxford) 2011;50:1424–30.

3. Takao M. Targeted therapy and progressive multifocal leukoencephalopathy (PML): PML in the era of monoclonal antibody therapies. *Brain Nerve* 2013;65:1363–74.

4. Lisnevskaia L, Murphy G, Isenberg D. Systemic lupus erythematosus. *Lancet* 2014;384:1878–88.

5. Murray E, Perry M. Off-label use of rituximab in systemic lupus erythematosus: a systematic review. *Clin Rheumatol* 2010;29:707–16.

6. Lu TY-T, Ng KP, Cambridge G, et al. A retrospective seven-year analysis of the use of B cell depletion therapy in systemic lupus erythematosus at University College London Hospital: the first fifty patients. *Arthritis Rheum* 2009;61:482–7.

7. Rosman Z, Shoenfeld Y, Zandman-Goddard G. Biologic therapy for autoimmune diseases: an update. *BMC Med* 2013;11:88.

8. Merrill J, Buyon J, Furie R, et al. Assessment of flares in lupus patients enrolled in a phase II/III study of rituximab (EXPLORER). *Lupus* 2011;20:709–16.

9. Rovin BH, Furie R, Latinis K, et al. Efficacy and safety of rituximab in patients with active proliferative lupus nephritis: the Lupus Nephritis Assessment with Rituximab study. *Arthritis Rheum* 2012;64:1215–26.

10. Ramos-Casals M, Soto MJ, Cuadrado MJ, Khamashta MA. Rituximab in systemic lupus erythematosus: A systematic review of off-label use in 188 cases. *Lupus* 2009;18:767–76.

11. Leandro MJ, Cambridge G, Edwards JC, Ehrenstein MR, Isenberg DA. B-cell depletion in the treatment of patients with systemic lupus erythematosus: a longitudinal analysis of 24 patients. *Rheumatology* 2005;44:1542–5.

12. Ezeonyeji AN, Isenberg DA. Early treatment with rituximab in newly diagnosed systemic lupus erythematosus patients: a steroid-sparing regimen. *Rheumatology* 2011;51:476–81.

13. Condon MB, Ashby D, Pepper RJ, et al. Prospective observational single-centre cohort study to evaluate the effectiveness of treating lupus nephritis with rituximab and mycophenolate mofetil but no oral steroids. *Ann Rheum Dis* 2013;72:1280–6.

14. Thornton CC, Ambrose N, Ioannou Y. Ofatumumab: A novel treatment for severe systemic lupus erythematosus. *Rheumatology* (Oxford). 2015;54:559–60.

15. Jordan N, Lutalo PMK, D'Cruz DP. Novel therapeutic agents in clinical development for systemic lupus erythematosus. *BMC Med* 2013;11:120.

16. Strand V, Petri M, Kalunian K, et al. Epratuzumab for patients with moderate to severe flaring SLE: health-related quality of life outcomes and corticosteroid use in the randomized controlled ALLEVIATE trials and extension study SL0006. *Rheumatology* (Oxford). 2014;53:502–11.

17. Wallace DJ, Kalunian K, Petri MA, et al. Efficacy and safety of epratuzumab in patients with moderate/severe active systemic lupus erythematosus: results from EMBLEM, a phase IIb, randomised, double-blind, placebo-controlled, multicentre study. *Ann Rheum Dis* 2014;73:183–90.

18. Navarra S V, Guzmán RM, Gallacher AE, et al. Efficacy and safety of belimumab in patients with active systemic lupus erythematosus: a randomised, placebo-controlled, phase 3 trial. *Lancet* 2011;377:721–31.

19. Van Vollenhoven RF, Petri MA, Cervera R, et al. Belimumab in the treatment of systemic lupus erythematosus: high disease activity predictors of response. *Ann Rheum Dis* 2012;71:1343–9.

20. Ginzler EM, Wallace DJ, Merrill JT, et al. Disease control and safety of belimumab plus standard therapy over 7 years in patients with systemic lupus erythematosus. *J Rheumatol* 2013;41:300–9.

21. Dall'Era M, Chakravarty E, Wallace D, et al. Reduced B lymphocyte and immunoglobulin levels after atacicept treatment in patients with systemic lupus erythematosus: results of a multicenter, phase Ib, double-blind, placebo-controlled, dose-escalating trial. *Arthritis Rheum* 2007;56:4142–50.

22. Isenberg D, Wofsy D, Li Y, et al. Pharmacodynamics and predictive biomarkers in patients treated with atacicept: data from the APRIL-SLE trial. *Arthritis Rheum* 2013;65(Suppl 10):2551.

23. Borba HHL, Wiens A, de Souza TT, Correr CJ, Pontarolo R. Efficacy and safety of biologic therapies for systemic lupus erythematosus treatment: systematic review and meta-analysis. *BioDrugs* 2013;28:211–28.

24. Cogollo E, Silva MA, Isenberg D. Profile of atacicept and its potential in the treatment of systemic lupus erythematosus. *Drug Des Devel Ther* Jan;9:1331–9.

25. Khamashta M, Merrill J, Werth V, et al. Safety and efficacy of sifalimumab, an anti IFN alpha monoclonal antibody, in a phase 2b study of moderate to severe systemic lupus erythematosus (SLE). *ACR Late-breaking Abstract Session*, 2014.

26. Kalunian K, Merrill J, Maciuca R, et al. A Phase II study of the efficacy and safety of rontalizumab (rhuMAb interferon-α) in patients with systemic lupus erythematosus (ROSE). *Ann Rheum Dis* 2015 June. doi:10.1136/annrheumdis-2014-206090.

27. Furie R, Nicholls K, Cheng T-T, et al. Efficacy and safety of abatacept in lupus nephritis: a twelve-month, randomized, double-blind study. *Arthritis Rheumatol* (Hoboken, NJ). 2014;66:379–89.

28. Wofsy D, Hillson JL, Diamond B. Comparison of alternative primary outcome measures for use in lupus nephritis clinical trials. *Arthritis Rheum* 2013;65:1586–91.

29. Kamal A, Khamashta M. The efficacy of novel B cell biologics as the future of SLE treatment: a review. *Autoimmun Rev* 2014;13:1094–101.

Chapter 8

Juvenile systemic lupus erythematosus

Claire Louise Murphy, Yiannis Ioannou, and Nicola Ambrose

> **Key points**
> - Juvenile SLE is a more aggressive disease than adult-onset SLE and has a higher mortality rate.
> - Macrophage activation syndrome is a potentially life-threatening complication of JSLE, which may mimic the underlying disease or be confused with sepsis.
> - Transferring care from paediatric to adult care can be a difficult milestone and should be tailored to the individual patient.

Introduction

Juvenile-onset systemic lupus erythematous (JSLE) is a chronic complex multisystem autoimmune disease, which represents 15–20% of all SLE cases.[1] Clinical presentation of JSLE is similar to adult-onset SLE, but there are some well-documented differences. JSLE is more aggressive, with more frequent renal and haematological manifestations. Mortality rates when corrected for age are higher than that of adult-onset SLE.[2] Infantile-onset SLE has a particularly high mortality rate.[3] The female to male ratio is approximately 5:1, lower than the 9:1 ratio in adult SLE.[4] Management of JSLE requires a multisystemic, holistic approach with recognition of psychosocial factors that occur during normal childhood and adolescence.

Epidemiology

JSLE prevalence ranges from approximately 40 cases per 100,000 in Caucasians to more than 200 cases per 100,000 among black people.[5] SLE is uncommon before puberty. However, the upper cut off age in JSLE studies has varied from 14 and 20 years of age and therefore comparison between juvenile data sets is difficult. Median age of onset is between 12–14 years and it is rare before 5 years of age.[6]

Pathophysiology

As with adult-onset SLE, the cause of JSLE is unknown. It appears to be multifactorial with genetic, immunological, hormonal, and environmental influences. All components of the immune system seem to be involved with dysregulation of the innate and adaptive systems.

Genetic susceptibility

Congenital complement deficiencies are present in about 1% of patients with JSLE;[7] the best characterized being C1q deficiency. The disease linked to homozygous C1q deficiency is best described as lupus-like with lower levels of antinuclear antibody (ANA) and double-stranded DNA (dsDNA) antibody positivity, and less renal and cerebral involvement.

Genetics play an important role in the pathogenesis of adult-onset SLE and JSLE. There is an approximate 25% concordance amongst monozygotic twins compared with 2% concordance in dizygotic twins in SLE.[8] The UK juvenile cohort study showed that 38% of patients with JSLE had a family history of at least one autoimmune disease.[9]

Genome-wide association studies (GWAS) are beginning to add further to our understanding of SLE with over 40 genes being implicated to date. Genes relating to pathways involved in the removal of anti-DNA-nucleosome complexes, such as complement, are among the strongest genetic risk factors.[10] Increased nuclear factor-kappaB (NF-κB) sensitivity has been identified, via a SLE susceptibility gene UBE2L3 (ubiquitination gene).[11]

Genetic overproduction of interferon-α, complement deficiencies, and apoptosis defects can lead to monogenic SLE.[12] New genetic techniques should lead to the discovery of new genes and help our understanding of the pathogenesis.

The immature immune system

Over-activity of the immune system appears to be a major factor in SLE with up-regulation of B cells, T cells, natural killer cells, monocytes, and dendritic cells. There are abnormalities in complement, in cytokine pathways, and in apoptosis.[13] Cytokines including interleukin-6 (IL-6), interleukin-10 (IL-10), interleukin 17 (IL-17), type I interferon (IFN), B lymphocyte stimulator (BLyS), and tumour necrosis factor-alpha (TNF-α) have all been implicated in SLE pathogenesis. Neutrophil extracellular traps (NETs) are fibrous networks of chromatin and antimicrobial factors that are released by neutrophils to trap and kill pathogens. Increased NET formation (NETosis) or insufficient degradation of NETs can promote autoimmunity due to the contents being exposed to the immune system.[14]

There are well described differences between the immune system in children and adults. Young children and infants appear to be more susceptible to infection. They also may have suboptimal responses to vaccines.[15] The total number of immune cells differs depending on age. In the first few months of life, helper T cells peak up to four times higher than in adults and then slowly decline reaching adult levels at around six years of age.[16] IgA levels are lower in infants than in adults. IgG1 and IgG3 reach 60% of adult levels at one year of age and IgG2 and IgG4 at 2–5 years of age.[15] Although some lymphocyte phenotypic differences have been described between young children and adults, very little is known about what functional changes occur at puberty across the innate and adaptive immune system that clearly lower the threshold for the development of JSLE.

Hormonal influences

Although adult-onset SLE affects a higher proportion of females, this is not as high in childhood SLE. One explanation for this is differences in oestrogen profiles. Oestrogen is known to affect the immune system via its oestrogen receptors (ERα and ERβ); and *ESR1* and *ESR2* genes encode these receptors. Oestrogens acting via receptors are important in the pathogenesis of SLE. The C variant of rs2234693, a single nucleotide polymorphism (SNP), increases transcription of *ESR1*. The T allele of this SNP was associated with early-onset SLE. A higher prevalence of the *ESR1* C allele among children with JSLE compared with controls suggests that increased activity of the oestrogen receptor is pathogenic. Allele A of the *ESR2* SNP (rs4986938) was associated with Adult SLE.[17] However, how puberty may affect oestrogen receptor expression, and how activation of oestrogen receptors may lower the threshold for lupus again remains unknown. In the Safety of Estrogens in Lupus Erythematosus National Assessment (SELENA) trial, the combined oral contraceptive pill did not increase the risk of SLE flare.[18]

The UK Juvenile-Onset SLE study group showed that male patients with JSLE were younger at presentation and were more likely to have a discoid rash compared with females. Males were less likely to have arthritis than females.[9] However, a recent review showed that there was no clear association between gender and mortality or disease activity in SLE.[19]

Environmental influences

UV radiation appears to play a role in the pathogenesis of SLE. There may be an association with low vitamin D levels and SLE. Drugs such as hydralazine, procainamide, and TNF-antagonists are risk factors for SLE. Infections have been implicated. Epstein–Barr virus antibodies have been found to be more prevalent in children and adolescents with JSLE compared with healthy controls (99% vs 70%).[20]

Clinical features with emphasis on differences between JSLE and adult SLE

Patients with JSLE display a wide range of clinical manifestations, which can fluctuate over time. Some may have mild lupus and others have life-threatening disease.

Systemic features

Fever and lymphadenopathy are more frequently observed in JSLE than in adult-onset SLE. Although Raynaud's is commonly seen in JSLE, it is more commonly seen in adult-onset SLE. Sicca symptoms are more common in adult-onset SLE.[21] It may be that younger patients have a greater reserve of salivary ducts and remain asymptomatic for longer. JSLE is more severe and has a worse prognosis than adult-onset SLE.[22] Please see Table 8.1.

Skin manifestations

A malar rash, and oral ulceration is more common in JSLE than in adult-onset SLE.[23] Alopecia is usually non-scarring and is more common in adults.[24] Discoid lesions and

Table 8.1 Key clinical differences between JSLE and adult-onset SLE		
Clinical features	Juvenile SLE	Adult-onset SLE
Fever	++	+
Lymphadenopathy	++	+
Raynaud's	+	++
Dry eyes	+	++
Butterfly rash	++	+
Alopecia	++	+
Oral ulceration	++	+
Arthralgia	+	++
Lupus nephritis	++	+
Neuropsychiatric	++	+
Livedo reticularis	+	++

subacute lupus are more frequently seen in adult-onset SLE.[23] Livedo reticularis is less common in JSLE.[24]

Musculoskeletal manifestations

The reporting of joint pains increases with advancing age. True arthritis may be more common in JSLE, whilst arthralgia and myalgia may be more frequent in adult-onset SLE.[25,26] Avascular necrosis is more common in children than in adults with lupus.[27]

Renal disease

Lupus nephritis is more common and severe in JSLE and is more often a presenting feature. As with adults, diffuse proliferative glomerulonephritis is the commonest histological diagnosis. Children may present with severe nephritic syndrome, hypertension, nephrotic range proteinuria, and oedema, but are more commonly asymptomatic.[26] One study showed that 47% of JSLE patients had evidence of renal involvement at presentation and 80% at the time of their last review.[9] Patients with JSLE are more likely to have dialysis compared with those with adult-onset SLE (19% vs 5.7%; $p < 0.001$).[28]

Neurological manifestations

Neuropsychiatric manifestations may be more common in JSLE (20–45%) compared with adult-onset SLE (10–25%).[5] However, it is difficult to quantify manifestations, as there is such a wide array, ranging from 15–90%, depending on diagnostic criteria and patient selection. For instance, headaches are frequent but the prevalence of true 'lupus headache' is unknown. It is imperative that all other aetiologies of neuropsychiatric disease are excluded prior to diagnosis. Psychosis with visual hallucinations is the commonest manifestation of neuropsychiatric disease associated with JSLE. Neuropsychiatric manifestations often occur within the first year of disease onset. Seizures are more prevalent in JSLE than in adult-onset SLE.[21,29] Mood disorders and headaches are frequent. Diagnosing true neuropsychiatric JSLE may be challenging in the adolescent patient, where rebellion and testing boundaries is part of normal development.

Haematological manifestations

Haemolytic anaemia and thrombocytopenia are more common in JSLE than in adult-onset SLE. Patients with a positive ANA and immune thrombocytopenic purpura (ITP) are at higher risk of developing autoimmune diseases such as SLE.[30]

Gastrointestinal manifestations

Abdominal pain is common in JSLE, and occasionally may be secondary to ascites, pancreatitis, autoimmune hepatitis, or intestinal vasculitis.[31] There is a greater prevalence of autoimmune liver disease (smooth muscle antibody-positive, biopsy proven) in JSLE compared with adult-onset SLE (9.8% vs 1.3%; $p < 0.001$).[32] Also liver disease preceded the diagnosis in many of those with JSLE but in none of the adults.[32]

Cardiopulmonary manifestations

Cardiopulmonary involvement is more common in adult-onset SLE than in JSLE.[33] Pleuritis is the most common feature in both groups. Pericarditis appears to be as common in JSLE and adult-onset SLE.[21] Pulmonary hypertension is rare in SLE.[34] Adult-onset SLE is associated with a 10-fold risk of coronary artery disease which is not explained by conventional risk factors.[35] One study of 157 patients with JSLE showed pericarditis in 28.7%, cardiomegaly in 33.8%, and arrhythmia/conduction defects in 12.7%.[34] Long-term follow-up studies are underway which will help evaluate the true cardiovascular risk in JSLE.

Macrophage activation syndrome and its treatment

Macrophage activation syndrome (MAS) is a potentially life-threatening condition which can complicate JSLE.[36] It is characterized by the infiltration of macrophages in bone marrow and in organs such as the liver, spleen, and lymph nodes. The pathogenesis is not fully understood, but it appears to be due to a defect in natural killer cells and cytokine dysregulation. Activation and uncontrolled proliferation of T lymphocytes and macrophages can lead to cytokine release and widespread haemophagocytosis. Infections (such as Epstein–Barr virus) and drugs may be a trigger. Patients may develop a high fever, headaches, fatigue, disorientation, seizures, and coma, and multisystem involvement may occur. Hyperferritinaemia is an important feature. Haematological features include pancytopenia, elevated liver enzymes, high triglycerides, high lactate dehydrogenase, and elevated D-dimers. Hyponatremia is frequently seen. The coagulation profile may show low fibrinogen, with prolongation of the prothrombin and partial thromboplastin time. Patients may develop purpura and bleed easily. Recognition of MAS in JSLE can be particularly challenging as it may mimic features of the underlying disease (eg, fever and cytopenias) or be confused with sepsis. Based on the HLH-94 protocol, treatment with high dose corticosteroids is necessary. Ciclosporin and etoposide are sometimes needed.[37]

Antiphospholipid syndrome

There are limited data on antiphospholipid syndrome (APS) in JSLE. The prevalence of antiphospholipid antibodies ranges from 27–66% for anticardiolipin antibodies and 24–62% for lupus anticoagulant.[38,39] Part of the problem is a lack of clarity with regards to classification of childhood onset APS, as the current classification criteria for APS include recurrent pregnancy loss as one of the clinical features that define disease.[40] Catastrophic antiphospholipid syndrome (CAPS) in paediatric patients is rare though very serious. One study showed that 10.3% of the 446 patients from the CAPS registry

Table 8.2 Key laboratory differences between JSLE and adult onset SLE

Haematology	Juvenile SLE	Adult-onset SLE
ANA	++	++
Anti-dsDNA	++	+
Anti-Ro	++	++
Anti-La	++	++
Anti-Smith	++	+
Anti-RNP	++	++
Rheumatoid factor	+	++
Anti-cardiolipin (IgG and IgM)	++	+
Lupus anticoagulant	++	+
Anti-ribosomal P	++	+
Low C3	++	+
Haemolytic anaemia	++	+
Thrombocytopenia	++	+
Urine		
Urinary cellular casts	++	+

ANA: antinuclear antibodies: dsDNA: double-stranded DNA.

were below 18 years of age. Of the paediatric patients with CAPS, 68.9% suffered from primary APS and 28.9% from SLE. There appeared to be a higher prevalence of infection as a precipitating factor for in the paediatric population (60.9% vs 26.8% in the adult population; $p<0.001$) and of peripheral vessel thrombosis (52.2% vs 34.3%; $p = 0.017$).[41] A study of 121 patients with paediatric APS showed that those with primary APS were younger and had a higher frequency of arterial events, whereas patients with APS associated with autoimmune disease were older and had a higher frequency of venous events.[42]

Immunological manifestations

Antinuclear antibodies are present in over 90% of patients with adult-onset SLE and JSLE.[33] There is a similar occurrence of anti-Ro and anti-La. It is more common to have high anti-dsDNA and low C3 in JSLE. Anti-histone and anti-ribosomal P antibodies are more common in JSLE.[43] Please see Table 8.2.

Treatment

A multidisciplinary approach is essential to ensure quality care for patients with JSLE. Patients should be treated in a specialist centre where related specialists are also available (eg, haematologists, nephrologists, neurologists). Involvement of the general practitioner, physiotherapist, occupational therapists, psychologists, play therapists, nurse specialists, social workers, and school teachers is key to ensuring optimal care.

Avoidance of UVA and UVB exposure is advised. Therefore patients with JSLE should avoid excessive sun and wear high factor sunscreen.

Early recognition and aggressive treatment is crucial in the management of JSLE in order to prevent irreversible damage. Due to the higher prevalence of renal and cerebral involvement, more intensive immunosuppression is usually required in JSLE.[44] Glucocorticoids are prescribed frequently with efforts to wean off as soon as possible. Children tend to have higher levels of glucocorticoids than adults, which contribute to damage, and may be a reason why children have an increased incidence of avascular necrosis compared with adults. Non-steroidal anti-inflammatory drugs (NSAIDs) are helpful for musculoskeletal disease but have significant side effects.

Mild/moderate JSLE

Hydroxychloroquine is helpful in skin and joint disease and can prevent flares of SLE. It inhibits toll-like receptors 7 and 9 and has effects on pro-inflammatory cytokines and reduces disease activity.[45] It also reduces low-density lipoprotein levels in SLE and appears to be cardioprotective.[46] There is also evidence to show that hydroxychloroquine is protective against thrombosis.[47] It is recommended for all patients with JSLE provided there are no contraindications.

Azathioprine (AZA) is a purine analogue that is used as a steroid-sparing agent in mild-moderate SLE, especially in patients who are having recurrent flares.

Methotrexate is useful in patients with lupus for musculoskeletal disease.

Renal/cerebral disease

Mycophenolate mofetil (MMF) is useful in lupus nephritis in JSLE like in adult-onset SLE.[48] MMF has been shown to be as effective for severe renal lupus (grades III and IV) as cyclophosphamide, and has fewer side effects.[49] The MAINTAIN nephritis trial compared MMF with azathioprine for long-term immunosuppression and reported that although there were fewer renal flares in the MMF group, this did not reach statistical significance. Therefore, both MMF and azathioprine are reasonably effective in maintaining remission;[50] however, data for JSLE is lacking.

Cyclophosphamide (500–750 mg/m^2 per month for six months, or the Euro-Lupus protocol of 500 mg fortnightly for 6 doses) is used only in severe JSLE, weighing up the future risks of infertility and malignancy. Cyclophosphamide is the preferred treatment in neuropsychiatric JSLE. Prepubertal girls seem to be protected from the gonadotoxic effects of cyclophosphamide.[51] The gonadotrophin releasing hormone (GnRH) analogue, triptorelin, is used for ovary protection in JSLE, and a recent randomized control trial has shown it to be effective in patients.[52] Gonadal functioning and preservation of reproductive function in JSLE has been explored but remains uncertain.[51,53,54]

B cell depletion

Rituximab is a chimeric anti-CD20 monoclonal antibody (MAB) and has been used successfully in patients with refractory JSLE.[55] Rituximab has been used in JSLE to treat immune thrombocytopenia purpura (ITP), autoimmune haemolytic anaemia, renal and neuropsychiatric JSLE and appears to be safe and efficacious. Despite failure of rituximab in the EXPLORER and LUNAR trials,[56,57] rituximab does appear to be efficacious and is widely used.[58] Novel anti-CD20 MABs may present novel options for patients allergic to rituximab. *Ocrelizumab* is a humanized CD20 antagonist which reached Phase III trials. However, the trial was stopped due to a large number of opportunistic infections. *Ofatumumab* is a human IgG1κ MAB that binds CD20 on B cells at a unique epitope. Although unlicensed, ofatumumab may be an effective alternative therapy for patients with SLE intolerant to rituximab (see Chapter 7).[59]

Belimumab is a MAB to the soluble human B lymphocyte stimulator (BLyS) protein and has been shown to be effective in adult-onset SLE (see Chapter 7) and was approved by the FDA in 2011. Clinical trials with belimumab in children with SLE are currently in progress.[60]

Epratuzumab is a human MAB that targets CD22 that was studied in phase III clinical trials and was considered promising in JSLE[61] until negative results were recently announced (see Chapter 7).

Other available treatments

Intravenous immune globulin (IVIG) and plasma exchange may been useful in acute life-threatening disease.

Stem cell transplantation may be used in patients with severe disease, unresponsive to other therapy.[62–64] One study showed that three of six severely ill patients (all female, age 15–29 years) with severe refractory SLE died post stem cell transplantation and three survived and remained in remission.[63] Stem cell transplantation is not widely used due to the potentially fatal side effects.

Specific adolescent concerns

Long-term prognosis has improved for patients with SLE with the 10-year survival rate now over 90%.[65,66] The emphasis is on maintaining health, preventing damage, achieving growth, and successfully transitioning from paediatric to adult care.

Access to care and delays in initial diagnosis are well reported in JSLE.[67] Patients treated early and aggressively have a better prognosis than those who have their treatment delayed. The UK JSLE cohort study showed that there is a wide variation in time to JSLE diagnosis. However, overall prognosis is improving and life expectancy is now much longer.

Transferring care from paediatric to adult clinics

Moving from the paediatric JSLE clinic to the adult SLE clinic can be a difficult milestone for children and parents. The transition is not a single event and should occur over several years. Research has shown that adolescents with rheumatic conditions rate their mental health, use of health services, and activities more negatively than those without chronic disease or with other chronic diseases.[68] Transition to adult care should be tailored to each individual patient.

School attendance, vocational planning

Adolescents with JSLE are at higher risk for delayed psychosocial and cognitive development than their peers. Additionally clinic appointments, medication monitoring blood tests, side effects, fatigue, and disease flare ups lead to reduced school attendance. A holistic approach needs to be taken in managing their individual needs, taking vocational planning and school attendance into consideration.

Self-management

As children grow up, they need to learn about their condition, medications, self-administration, and monitoring requirements. Adolescents may respond to a problem-solving approach rather than a paternalistic approach.

Bone health

Osteopenia affects approximately 40% of those with JSLE.[69] Vertebral fractures occur in up to 10% of patients. Patients should ensure sufficient intake of vitamin D and calcium to prevent osteopenia or osteoporosis. Weight-bearing exercise is crucial in maintaining bone strength. Bisphosphonates have a long half-life and are potentially teratogenic so ideally should be avoided in adolescents. Dual-energy X-ray absorptiometry (DXA) use in children is controversial but it is generally recommended at the time of diagnosis and every two years thereafter.

Growth

Growth failure occurs in approximately 15% of patients with JSLE and therefore regular measurement of height and weight is essential. Active disease, corticosteroids, and concomitant autoimmune disease such as thyroid disease may result in short stature. Growth hormone in JSLE may result in increased disease flares.[70] Early referral to endocrinology is recommended as soon as growth failure is apparent.

Cardiovascular health

Like adults with SLE, patients with JSLE have an increased cardiovascular risk. Atherosclerosis begins early in life even in healthy children. Risk factors such as dyslipidaemia, high blood pressure and glucose, smoking, and lack of exercise should be addressed. Aspirin and hydroxychloroquine should be considered in JSLE especially if antiphospholipid antibody positive. Schanberg et al. studied the use of atorvastatin over three years in JSLE and there was no statistically significant benefit.[71] The APPLE (Atherosclerosis Prevention in Pediatric Lupus Erythematosus) study suggests atorvastatin may reduce atherosclerosis progression in pubertal patients with SLE with higher C-reactive protein. Further research in this area is needed.[72]

Malignancy

Little is known regarding the risk of malignancy in JSLE. The risk of non-Hodgkin's lymphoma appears to be increased in adult-onset SLE.[73] A cohort study of 1020 juvenile patients aged under 18 years, were observed for an average of 7.8 patient years. Two patients developed non-Hodgkin's lymphoma and one patient had leukaemia. The non-haematological cancers included one bladder, one breast, one thyroid and one brain, three head and neck and four non-specified cancers. Although this study showed an increased malignancy risk in patients with JSLE compared with the general population, this translated to a relatively low absolute risk (1.75 cancers per 1000 patient years). The risk may be higher after patients have transferred to adult care.[74] Longer term studies are required.

Vaccinations

Patients with JSLE are at increased risk of infection. Annual influenza vaccine and 5-yearly pneumococcal vaccines are recommended. There is an increased risk of cervical intraepithelial neoplasia (CIN) in SLE.[75] Adolescent girls should receive human papilloma vaccine and have regular cervical smears. Live vaccinations are contraindicated while on immunosuppressant therapy and for three months after discontinuation.

Fertility and contraception

Active disease is associated with delayed menarche, amenorrhoea, or oligomenorrhoea. Oestrogen-based contraception is contraindicated in patients with APS associated with JSLE, because of a risk of thrombosis. However, in those without antiphospholipid antibodies, the combined oral contraceptive pill may be prescribed.[76]

Medication toxicity

High-dose steroids may lead to premature atherosclerosis, secondary osteoporosis, and glucose intolerance. In adolescence, obesity, growth delay, hirsutism, and striae may have a significant impact for body image and lead to poor adherence.

Research

Performing clinical trials is curtailed in JSLE due to the small number of eligible patients and due to the heterogeneity of the disease. To date, treatments have been based on those used in adult-onset SLE. Patients with rheumatic disease, regardless of their age, should have the opportunity to participate in research. PRINTO (Paediatric Rheumatology International Trials Organisation) is a non-governmental international research network, which includes 59 countries with the goal to conduct international clinical trials and outcome studies in children with rheumatic diseases.[77]

Measurement of disease activity is crucial, especially now that various biologics are undergoing clinical trials. The BILAG (British Isles lupus assessment group) index, SLEDAI (systemic lupus erythematosus disease activity index) and SLAM (systemic lupus activity measure) indices are validated for use in JSLE.[78] The BILAG-2004 index is based on the physician's intention to treat and has been shown to measure SLE disease activity better than the SLEDAI-2000.[79]

The BILAG index was adapted for use in JSLE,[80] and subsequently used in the UK juvenile SLE cohort study and was named the paediatric BILAG (pBILAG). The pBILAG index collects more detailed information about organ-related disease activity than that incorporated within the American College of Rheumatology (ACR) criteria.[81] However, this index was designed for adults with lupus so may not capture the full spectrum of disease.

New biomarkers

Novel biomarkers would help in identifying JSLE, disease monitoring, and prediction of flares.[82] There has been much interest in looking for novel biomarkers for SLE and JSLE. Those published include monocyte chemoattractant protein-1/CCL-2, neutrophil gelantinase-associated lipocalin, urine protein signature, and colony-stimulating factor 1.

Other biomarkers being investigated in JSLE include microRNA, type 1 interferon, cell adhesion molecules, and complement components. Recent studies show that complement split products may be better than the traditional C3 and C4. Circulating erythrocyte E-C4d levels appeared higher in patients with lupus nephritis compared with healthy controls.[83]

Conclusion

JSLE is similar to adult-onset SLE, but there are distinct differences in clinical features, serology, and management requirements. It is more aggressive, with a higher prevalence of renal manifestations requiring high-dose immunosuppression. Obesity, growth delay, and psychological effects of both the disease and treatments can pose major problems in the management of children and adolescents. A holistic, multidisciplinary approach is necessary. Patients need support so that they can live a full life despite having a chronic debilitating disease. International collaboration and further research is needed to optimize care for these patients.

References

1. Mina R, Brunner HI. Pediatric lupus: are there differences in presentation, genetics, response to therapy, and damage accrual compared with adult lupus? *Rheum Dis Clin North Am* 2010:36;53–80,vii–viii.

2. Amaral B, Murphy G, Ioannou Y, Isenberg DA. A comparison of the outcome of adolescent and adult-onset systemic lupus erythematosus. *Rheumatology* (Oxford), 2014:53;1130–5.

3. Zulian F, Pluchinotta F, Martini G, Da Dalt L, Zacchello G. Severe clinical course of systemic lupus erythematosus in the first year of life. *Lupus* 2008:17;780–6.

4. Lo JT, Tsai MJ, Wang LH, et al. Sex differences in pediatric systemic lupus erythematosus: a retrospective analysis of 135 cases. *J Microbiol Immunol Infect* 1999:32;173–8.

5. Papadimitraki ED, Isenberg DA. Childhood- and adult-onset lupus: an update of similarities and differences. *Expert Rev Clin Immunol* 2009:5;391–403.

6. Brunner HI, Huggins J, Klein-Gitelman MS. Pediatric SLE: towards a comprehensive management plan. *Nat Rev Rheumatol* 2011:7;225–33.

7. Pickering MC, Walport MJ. Links between complement abnormalities and systemic lupus erythematosus. *Rheumatology* (Oxford) 2000:39;133–41.

8. Sullivan KE. Genetics of systemic lupus erythematosus. Clinical implications. *Rheum Dis Clin North Am* 2000:26;229–56,v–vi.

9. Watson L, Leone V, Pilkington C, et al. Disease activity, severity, and damage in the UK Juvenile-Onset Systemic Lupus Erythematosus Cohort. *Arthritis Rheum* 2012;64;2356–65.

10. Azevedo PC, Murphy G, Isenberg DA. Pathology of systemic lupus erythematosus: the challenges ahead. *Methods Mol Biol* 2014:1134;1–16.

11. Lewis MJ, Vyse S, Shields AM et al. UBE2L3 Polymorphism Amplifies NF-kappaB activation and promotes plasma cell development, linking linear ubiquitination to multiple autoimmune diseases. *Am J Hum Genet* 2015:96;221–34.

12. Belot A, Cimaz R. Monogenic forms of systemic lupus erythematosus: new insights into SLE pathogenesis. *Pediatr Rheumatol Online J* 2012:10;21.

13. Gualtierotti R, Biggioggero M, Penatti AE, Meroni PL. Updating on the pathogenesis of systemic lupus erythematosus. *Autoimmun Rev* 2010:10;3–7.

14. Midgley A, Watson L, Beresford MW. New insights into the pathogenesis and management of lupus in children. *Arch Dis Child* 2014:99;563–7.

15. Tobin NH, Aldrovandi GM. Immunology of pediatric HIV infection. *Immunol Rev* 2013: 254;143–69.

16. Shearer WT, Rosenblatt HM, Gelman RS, et al. Lymphocyte subsets in healthy children from birth through 18 years of age: the Pediatric AIDS Clinical Trials Group P1009 study. *J Allergy Clin Immunol* 2003:112;973–80.

17. Kisiel BM, Kosinska J, Wierzbowska M, et al. Differential association of juvenile and adult systemic lupus erythematosus with genetic variants of oestrogen receptors alpha and beta. *Lupus* 2011:20;85–9.

18. Petri M, Kim MY, Kalunian KC, et al. Combined oral contraceptives in women with systemic lupus erythematosus. *N Engl J Med* 2005:353;2550–8.

19. Murphy G, Isenberg D. Effect of gender on clinical presentation in systemic lupus erythematosus. *Rheumatology* (Oxford) 2013:52;2108–15.

20. James JA, Kaufman KM, Farris AD, Taylor-Albert E, Lehman TJ, Harley JB. An increased prevalence of Epstein-Barr virus infection in young patients suggests a possible etiology for systemic lupus erythematosus. *J Clin Invest* 1997:100;3019–26.

21. Livingston B, Bonner A, Pope J. Differences in clinical manifestations between childhood-onset lupus and adult-onset lupus: a meta-analysis. *Lupus* 2011:20;1345–55.

22. Carreno L, Lopez-Longo FJ, Monteagudo I, et al. Immunological and clinical differences between juvenile and adult onset of systemic lupus erythematosus. *Lupus* 1999:8;287–92.

23. Tarr T, Dérfalvi B, Győri N, et al. Similarities and differences between pediatric and adult patients with systemic lupus erythematosus. *Lupus* 2015:24;796–803.

24. Chiewchengchol D, Murphy R, Edwards SW, Beresford MW. Mucocutaneous manifestations in juvenile-onset systemic lupus erythematosus: a review of literature. *Pediatr Rheumatol Online J* 2015:13;1.

25. Font J, Cervera R, Espinosa G, et al. Systemic lupus erythematosus (SLE) in childhood: analysis of clinical and immunological findings in 34 patients and comparison with SLE characteristics in adults. *Ann Rheum Dis* 1998:57;456–9.

26. Morgan TA, Watson L, McCann LJ, Beresford MW. Children and adolescents with SLE: not just little adults. *Lupus* 2013:22;1309–19.

27. White PH. Pediatric systemic lupus erythematosus and neonatal lupus. *Rheum Dis Clin North Am* 1994:20;119–27.

28. Tucker LB, Uribe AG, Fernandez M, et al. Adolescent onset of lupus results in more aggressive disease and worse outcomes: results of a nested matched case–control study within LUMINA, a multiethnic US cohort (LUMINA LVII). *Lupus* 2008:17;314–22.

29. Yu HH, Lee JH, Wang LC, Yang YH, Chiang BL. Neuropsychiatric manifestations in pediatric systemic lupus erythematosus: a 20-year study. *Lupus* 2006:15;651–7.

30. Zimmerman SA, Ware RE. Clinical significance of the antinuclear antibody test in selected children with idiopathic thrombocytopenic purpura. *J Pediatr Hematol Oncol* 1997:19;297–303.

31. Richer O, Ulinski T, Lemelle I, et al. Abdominal manifestations in childhood-onset systemic lupus erythematosus. *Ann Rheum Dis* 2007:66;174–8.

32. Irving KS, Sen D, Tahir H, et al. A comparison of autoimmune liver disease in juvenile and adult populations with systemic lupus erythematosus-a retrospective review of cases. *Rheumatology* (Oxford) 2007:46;1171–3.

33. Tucker LB, Menon S, Schaller JG, et al. Adult- and childhood-onset systemic lupus erythematosus: a comparison of onset, clinical features, serology, and outcome. *Br J Rheumatol* 1995:34;866–72.

34. Yeh TT, Yang YH, Lin YT, et al. Cardiopulmonary involvement in pediatric systemic lupus erythematosus: a twenty-year retrospective analysis. *J Microbiol Immunol Infect* 2007:40;525–31.

35. Rahman P, Aguero S, Gladman DD, Hallett D, Urowitz MB. Contribution of traditional risk factors to coronary artery disease in patients with systemic lupus erythematosus. *J Rheumatol* 1999:26;2363–8.

36. Pringe A, Trail L, Ruperto N, et al. Macrophage activation syndrome in juvenile systemic lupus erythematosus: an under-recognized complication? *Lupus* 2007:16;587–92.

37. Trottestam H, Horne AC, Aricó M, et al. Chemoimmunotherapy for hemophagocytic lymphohistiocytosis: long-term results of the HLH-94 treatment protocol. Blood 2011:118;4577–84.

38. Seaman DE, Londino AV Jr, Kwoh CK, et al. Antiphospholipid antibodies in pediatric systemic lupus erythematosus. *Pediatrics* 1995:96;1040–5.

39. Berube C, Mitchell L, David M, et al. The relationship of antiphospholipid antibodies to thromboembolic events in pediatric patients with systemic lupus erythematosus: a cross-sectional study. *Pediatr Res* 1998:44;351–6.

40. Miyakis S, Lockshin MD, Atsumi T, et al. International consensus statement on an update of the classification criteria for definite antiphospholipid syndrome (APS). *J Thromb Haemost* 2006:4;295–306.

41. Berman H, Rodríguez-Pintó I, Cervera R, et al. Pediatric catastrophic antiphospholipid syndrome: descriptive analysis of 45 patients from the 'CAPS Registry'. *Autoimmun Rev* 2014:13;157–62.

42. Avcin T, Cimaz R, Silverman ED, et al. Pediatric antiphospholipid syndrome: clinical and immunologic features of 121 patients in an international registry. *Pediatrics* 2008:122;e1100–7.

43. Hoffman IE, Lauwerys BR, De Keyser F, et al. Juvenile-onset systemic lupus erythematosus: different clinical and serological pattern than adult-onset systemic lupus erythematosus. *Ann Rheum Dis* 2009:68;412–15.

44. Hersh AO, von Scheven E, Yazdany J, et al. Differences in long-term disease activity and treatment of adult patients with childhood- and adult-onset systemic lupus erythematosus. *Arthritis Rheum* 2009:61;13–20.

45. Willis R, Seif AM, McGwin G Jr, et al. Effect of hydroxychloroquine treatment on pro-inflammatory cytokines and disease activity in SLE patients: data from LUMINA (LXXV), a multiethnic US cohort. *Lupus* 2012:21;830–5.

46. Cairoli E, Rebella M, Danese N, Garra V, Borba EF. Hydroxychloroquine reduces low-density lipoprotein cholesterol levels in systemic lupus erythematosus: a longitudinal evaluation of the lipid-lowering effect. *Lupus* 2012:21;1178–82.

47. Ruiz-Irastorza G, Egurbide MV, Pijoan JI, et al. Effect of antimalarials on thrombosis and survival in patients with systemic lupus erythematosus. *Lupus* 2006:15;577–83.

48. Kazyra I, Pilkington C, Marks SD, Tullus K. Mycophenolate mofetil treatment in children and adolescents with lupus. *Arch Dis Child* 2010;95;1059–61.

49. Appel AS, Appel GB. An update on the use of mycophenolate mofetil in lupus nephritis and other primary glomerular diseases. *Nat Clin Pract Nephrol* 2009:5;132–42.

50. Houssiau FA, D'Cruz D, Sangle S, et al. Azathioprine versus mycophenolate mofetil for long-term immunosuppression in lupus nephritis: results from the MAINTAIN Nephritis Trial. *Ann Rheum Dis* 2010:69;2083–9.

51. Silva CA, Leal MM, Leone C, et al. Gonadal function in adolescents and young women with juvenile systemic lupus erythematosus. *Lupus* 2002;11;419–25.

52. Brunner HI, Silva CA, Reiff A, et al. Randomized double-blinded dose escalation trial of triptorelin for ovary protection in childhood-onset systemic lupus erythematosus. *Arthritis Rheumatol* 2015:67;1377–85.

53. Silva CA, Brunner HI. Gonadal functioning and preservation of reproductive fitness with juvenile systemic lupus erythematosus. *Lupus* 2007;16;593–9.

54. Silva CA, Hallak J, Pasqualotto FF, et al. Gonadal function in male adolescents and young males with juvenile onset systemic lupus erythematosus. *J Rheumatol* 2002:29;2000–5.

55. Podolskaya A, Stadermann M, Pilkington C, et al. B cell depletion therapy for 19 patients with refractory systemic lupus erythematosus. *Arch Dis Child* 2008;93;401–6.

56. Merrill J, Buyon J, Furie R, et al. Assessment of flares in lupus patients enrolled in a phase II/III study of rituximab (EXPLORER). *Lupus* 2011:20;709–16.

57. Rovin BH, Furie R, Latinis K, et al. Efficacy and safety of rituximab in patients with active proliferative lupus nephritis: the Lupus Nephritis Assessment with Rituximab study. *Arthritis Rheum* 2012:64;1215–26.

58. Hickman RA, Hira-Kazal R, Yee CS, et al. The efficacy and safety of rituximab in a chart review study of 15 patients with systemic lupus erythematosus. *Clin Rheumatol* 2015:34;263–271.

59. Thornton CC, Ambrose N, Ioannou Y. Ofatumumab: a novel treatment for severe systemic lupus erythematosus. *Rheumatology* (Oxford), 2015. 54(3);559–60.

60. Furie R, Petri M, Zamani O, et al. A phase III, randomized, placebo-controlled study of belimumab, a monoclonal antibody that inhibits B lymphocyte stimulator, in patients with systemic lupus erythematosus. *Arthritis Rheum* 2011:63;3918–30.

61. Wallace DJ, Kalunian K, Petri MA, et al. Efficacy and safety of epratuzumab in patients with moderate/severe active systemic lupus erythematosus: results from EMBLEM, a phase IIb, randomised, double-blind, placebo-controlled multicentre study. *Ann Rheum Dis* 2014:73;183–90.

62. Farge D, Labopin M, Tyndall A, et al. Autologous hematopoietic stem cell transplantation for autoimmune diseases: an observational study on 12 years' experience from the European Group for Blood and Marrow Transplantation Working Party on Autoimmune Diseases. *Haematologica* 2010:95;284–92.

63. Lisukov IA, Sizikova SA, Kulagin AD, et al. High-dose immunosuppression with autologous stem cell transplantation in severe refractory systemic lupus erythematosus. *Lupus* 2004:13;89–94.

64. Milanetti F, Abinun M, Voltarelli JC, Burt RK. Autologous hematopoietic stem cell transplantation for childhood autoimmune disease. *Pediatr Clin North Am* 2010;57;239–71.

65. Cervera R, Abarca-Costalago M, Abramovicz D, et al. European Working Party on Systemic Lupus Erythematosus: a 10 year report. *Lupus* 2001:10;892–4.

66. Abu-Shakra M, Urowitz MB, Gladman DD, Gough J. Mortality studies in systemic lupus erythematosus. Results from a single center. II. Predictor variables for mortality. *J Rheumatol* 1995:22;1265–70.

67. Smith EM, Foster HE, Gray WK, Taylor-Robinson D, Beresford MW; UK JSLE Study Group. Predictors of access to care in juvenile systemic lupus erythematosus: evidence from the UK JSLE Cohort Study. *Rheumatology* (Oxford) 2014:53;557–61.

68. McDonagh JE, Shaw KL. Adolescent rheumatology transition care in the UK. *Pediatr Ann* 2012: 41;e8–15.

69. Lilleby V, Lien G, Frey Froslie K, Haugen M, Flato B, Forre O. Frequency of osteopenia in children and young adults with childhood-onset systemic lupus erythematosus. *Arthritis Rheum* 2005:52;2051–9.

70. Yap HK, Loke KY, Murugasu B, Lee BW. Subclinical activation of lupus nephritis by recombinant human growth hormone. *Pediatr Nephrol* 1998:12;133–5.

71. Schanberg LE, Sandborg C, Barnhart HX, et al. Use of atorvastatin in systemic lupus erythematosus in children and adolescents. *Arthritis Rheum* 2012:64;285–96.

72. Ardoin SP, Schanberg LE, Sandborg CI, Barnhart HX, Evans GW, Yow E, et al. Secondary analysis of APPLE study suggests atorvastatin may reduce atherosclerosis progression in pubertal lupus patients with higher C reactive protein. *Ann Rheum Dis* 2014:73;557–66.

73. Bernatsky S, Boivin Jf, Joseph L, et al. An international cohort study of cancer in systemic lupus erythematosus. *Arthritis Rheum* 2005:52;1481–90.

74. Bernatsky S, Clarke AE, Labrecque J, et al. Cancer risk in childhood-onset systemic lupus. *Arthritis Res Ther* 2013:15;R198.

75. Ognenovski VM, Marder W, Somers EC, et al. Increased incidence of cervical intraepithelial neoplasia in women with systemic lupus erythematosus treated with intravenous cyclophosphamide. *J Rheumatol* 2004:31;1763–7.

76. Lateef A, Petri M. Hormone replacement and contraceptive therapy in autoimmune diseases. *J Autoimmun* 2012:38;J170–6.

77. Ruperto N, Ravelli A, Cuttica R, et al. The Pediatric Rheumatology International Trials Organization criteria for the evaluation of response to therapy in juvenile systemic lupus erythematosus: prospective validation of the disease activity core set. *Arthritis Rheum* 2005:52;2854–64.

78. Gladman DD, Goldsmith CH, Urowitz MB, et al. Crosscultural validation and reliability of 3 disease activity indices in systemic lupus erythematosus. *J Rheumatol* 1992:19;608–11.

79. Yee CS, Isenberg DA, Prabu A, et al. BILAG-2004 index captures systemic lupus erythematosus disease activity better than SLEDAI-2000. *Ann Rheum Dis* 2008;67;873–6.

80. Marks SD, Pilkington C, Woo P, Dillon MJ. The use of the British Isles Lupus Assessment Group (BILAG) index as a valid tool in assessing disease activity in childhood-onset systemic lupus erythematosus. *Rheumatology* (Oxford) 2004:43;1186–9.

81. Chiewchengchol D, Murphy R, Edwards SW, Beresford MW. Mucocutaneous manifestations in a UK national cohort of juvenile-onset systemic lupus erythematosus patients. *Rheumatology* (Oxford) 2014:53;1504–12.

82. Abulaban KM, Brunner HI. Biomarkers for childhood-onset systemic lupus erythematosus. *Curr Rheumatol Rep* 2015:17;471.

83. Batal I, Liang K, Bastacky S, et al. Prospective assessment of C4d deposits on circulating cells and renal tissues in lupus nephritis: a pilot study. *Lupus* 2012:21;13–26.

Chapter 9

Management of special situations in systemic lupus erythematosus

April Jorge and Rosalind Ramsey-Goldman

> **Key points**
>
> - Most women with systemic lupus erythematosus (SLE) can have normal pregnancies. However, pregnant women with SLE have a higher risk of pre-eclampsia, premature labour, and spontaneous miscarriage compared with healthy peers.
> - Maternal and fetal risks associated with pregnancy are higher when SLE disease activity is poorly controlled prior to conception, particularly with active lupus nephritis.
> - Neonatal lupus can occur when pregnant women have the autoantibodies SSA/Ro and SSB/La. This syndrome can include congenital heart block, neonatal hepatitis, and a neonatal rash. Women with these autoantibodies should undergo prenatal monitoring, and hydroxychloroquine may be protective.
> - Normal pregnancy changes, which can include mild proteinuria, thrombocytopenia, and anaemia and chloasma, must be distinguished from an SLE flare.
> - There are multiple considerations in choosing methods of contraception for women with SLE. Intrauterine devices are the safest option, and women with increased risk of thrombosis, such as those with anti-phospholipid antibodies, should avoid oestrogen-containing contraceptives.
> - During pregnancy, the potential fetal risks of medications must be weighed against the need to control SLE disease activity.
> - Patients with SLE have an increased risk of premature cardiovascular disease (CVD). Multiple factors contribute to this increased risk including medication effects (particularly from corticosteroids), an increase in traditional cardiovascular risk factors, and inflammation from SLE.
> - Patients with SLE have an increased risk of osteoporosis, which is attributed to glucocorticoid use and the use of other medications that decrease bone density, as well as an increased incidence of vitamin D deficiency. Patients taking long-term glucocorticoids should receive calcium and vitamin D supplementation.
> - Patient with SLE should receive appropriate vaccinations, but live vaccines should not be given to those who are moderately immunosuppressed.
> - Patients with SLE have an increased risk of malignancy, including certain cancers such as non-Hodgkin's lymphoma, and cervical cancer. They should receive age-appropriate cancer screening.

Pregnancy in SLE

Introduction

Managing issues of pregnancy and fertility in systemic lupus erythematosus (SLE) remains a challenging and important aspect of caring for patients with SLE. A high proportion of SLE patients are females of childbearing age. Women with SLE generally have normal fertility. However, women with SLE have fewer live births than those without SLE. Systemic lupus erythematosus is associated with increased maternal and fetal risks during pregnancy, but most women with SLE will be able to have successful pregnancies.

Conception planning and counselling in SLE

The maternal and fetal risks associated with pregnancy are significantly improved when SLE disease activity is well controlled before conception. However, many medications used in the treatment of SLE can be teratogenic, as seen in Tables 9.1 and 9.2. Therefore, patients should be counselled on contraception use and the timing of pregnancy to occur when SLE disease activity is low, and the risk of teratogenicity from medications can be limited. Patients with a recent SLE flare (particularly within the past 4–6 months) are at higher risk for adverse pregnancy outcomes. The presence of antiphospholipid antibodies also increases the risks of pregnancy complications.

Under certain circumstances pregnancy should be deferred or avoided, and patients should be counselled as such. Women with pulmonary hypertension, interstitial lung disease, myocardial infarction, severe heart valve disorders, heart failure, and chronic kidney disease (creatinine >0.02 g/L or greater than 0.5 g/day protein-uria) are at particularly high risk. They may not be able to adequately compensate for the physiological changes of pregnancy including a 50% increase of plasma volume. Chronic kidney disease and pulmonary hypertension are also associated with endothelial dysfunction, which contributes to the increased risk for pre-eclampsia and placental insufficiency. Women who have had severe SLE flares and have been receiving highly teratogenic medications, such as mycophenolate mofetil or cyclophosphamide, should also be advised to avoid pregnancy until maternal disease is controlled on medications that are safer in pregnancy. See Table 9.1 for additional medication safety information in pregnancy and lactation. Controlled maternal disease for at least 6 months and the use of appropriate medications is recommended at time of conception.

Maternal and fetal morbidity in pregnant women with SLE

Pregnant women with SLE are at higher risk for pregnancy complications. One underlying mechanism for these complications is placental insufficiency that can occur due to inflammation and endothelial dysfunction. Women with SLE have a greater risk of undergoing spontaneous abortion than healthy pregnant women. When SLE activity is high during pregnancy there is up to 25% risk of pregnancy loss. However, with minimal disease activity, the risk approaches that of healthy pregnant women without SLE. Similarly, pregnant women with SLE are more likely than healthy controls to undergo premature labour, Caesarean delivery, and pre-eclampsia, and this risk is augmented by higher SLE disease activity, particularly when this involves active SLE nephritis. Women with active lupus nephritis are

Table 9.1 Safety and efficacy of pharmacotherapy for SLE during pregnancy and lactation: disease modifying anti-rheumatic drugs (DMARDs)				
Medication	Fetal effects	Recommendations	Use in lactation	Other comments
Hydroxychloroquine	Very rare congenital anomalies reported, not clearly due to drug	Generally recommended to continue through pregnancy	Yes	Long-acting so if patient wishes to avoid exposure during pregnancy, must discontinue at least 3–6 months before conception. If conception occurs while taking this medication, there is no benefit to discontinuing its use. May have benefits including reducing risk of neonatal lupus.
Methotrexate	Abortifacient; multiple congenital anomalies in surviving fetus	Contraindicated during pregnancy	No	Must discontinue 3–6 months before conception. Important to take folic acid supplementation.
Azathioprine	Rare neonatal immunosuppression and intrauterine growth restriction	Continue during pregnancy at dose up to 2 mg/kg/day if needed to control maternal disease	Yes	Fetal liver lacks ability to convert azathioprine to active metabolite 6-MP, so fetus should theoretically be protected from adverse effects.
Cyclophosphamide	Spontaneous abortion, congenital anomalies	Avoid unless maternal disease is life-threatening	No	Risk of future infertility for women with exposure to this medication, and risk increases with cumulative dose.
Mycophenolate	First trimester spontaneous abortion, multiple congenital anomalies	Avoid unless maternal disease is life-threatening during pregnancy. Use alternative agent if planning pregnancy.	No	Discontinue this medication at least 6 months prior to planned conception and switch to another drug if needed to control disease. Women of childbearing potential who are taking this medication must be monitored with periodic pregnancy tests during treatment.
Ciclosporin	May increase risk for premature birth, may cause congenital anomalies	Avoid use if possible, but weigh risks of maternal disease. Can continue at lowest possible dose with close monitoring.	No	Formulations often contain alcohol.

(continued)

Table 9.1 Continued

Medication	Fetal effects	Recommendations	Use in lactation	Other comments
Sulfasalazine	Risk of neonatal neutropenia at higher doses	Can continue through pregnancy, but limit doses to up to 2 g/day	Yes in healthy infants	Continue adequate folic acid supplementation with this medication.
Leflunomide	Multiple congenital anomalies and risk for spontaneous abortion	Avoid use for two years prior to conception or cholestyramine washout should be given. Must document negative plasma drug levels before planning pregnancy	No	Long half-life, with serum levels lasting up to 2 years. Can use cholestyramine to bind the medication for accelerated clearance.
Belimumab	Limited data, no known adverse fetal effects in humans	Avoid use during pregnancy and for 4 months prior to conception if possible, weighing risk of active maternal disease	No	Very limited data. This medication does likely cross the placenta so has potential for fetal effects.

Table 9.2 Safety and efficacy of pharmacotherapy during pregnancy and lactation: other commonly used medications in SLE

	Medication	Fetal effects	Recommendations	Use in lactation	Other comments
Anti-inflammatories	Non-steroidal anti-inflammatory drugs (NSAIDs)	Early exposure—rare cardiac anomalies and intrauterine growth retardation. Late (3rd trimester) exposure—premature closure of ductus arteriosus	Avoid if possible during pregnancy, particularly after 30 weeks	Caution	Breastfeeding immediately before a dose of NSAIDs can help minimize fetal exposure
	Glucocorticoids	Possible association of oral clefts, intrauterine growth restriction, and premature delivery, but these findings may be related to maternal disease rather than the glucocorticoids	Avoid high doses in 1st trimester, and use lowest effective dose possible. Use non-fluorinated steroids to avoid fetal effects	Yes	Fluorinated glucocorticoids are not metabolized by the placenta and have fetal effects; whereas non-fluorinated glucocorticoids are inactivated by 11- β-hydroxysteroid dehydrogenase
Antiplatelet	Aspirin	Very rare congenital anomalies	Low dose aspirin (<325 mg daily) can be used during pregnancy if benefits outweigh risks, such as in APS and prevention of pre-eclampsia	Caution	There is a risk for bleeding complications during delivery if high dose aspirin is continued at end of pregnancy
Anticoagulants	Heparin (unfractionated and LMWH)	None	Safe during pregnancy	Yes	Anticoagulant of choice during pregnancy. May increase risk of osteoporosis.
	Warfarin	CNS anomalies, limb hypoplasia, spontaneous abortion	Avoid during pregnancy	Yes—does not enter breast milk	Can be considered in cases of mechanical heart valves
	Target-specific oral anticoagulants (Xa inhibitors and direct thrombin inhibitors)	May increase risk of bleeding complications, possible congenital anomalies	Do not use during pregnancy—switch to LMWH	No	Limited data of these newer agents

(continued)

Table 9.2 Continued

Medication		Fetal effects	Recommendations	Use in lactation	Other comments
Anti-hypertensives	Angiotensin converting enzyme (ACE) inhibitors/ angiotensin receptor blockers	Fetal renal damage, oligohydramnios, lung hypoplasia	Contraindicated during pregnancy especially in 2nd and 3rd trimester	No	Fetal risks are higher in 2nd and 3rd trimester
	Methyldopa	No known adverse effects	Safe during pregnancy	Yes	Preferred agent in pregnancy
	Hydralazine	Craniofacial abnormalities in animals, not seen in humans	Considered safe during pregnancy	Caution—does enter breast milk	No high quality data, but has been standard of care to use during pregnancy
	Beta blockers	Intrauterine growth restriction	Avoid use in pregnancy, except in rare circumstances	Caution—does enter breast milk	Other anti-hypertensives are preferred
	Calcium channel blockers	Intrauterine growth restriction in animal studies	Considered safe during pregnancy	No	Can be used for hypertension and for Raynaud's syndrome
Statins (HMG coA reductase inhibitors)	All drugs in this class currently considered equivalent pregnancy risk	Rare reports of neural tube defects, oral clefts, congenital heart defects, intrauterine growth restriction	Avoid during pregnancy. Short discontinuation of these medications during pregnancy should not have long-term adverse maternal effects	No	Human studies inconclusive if risk of malformations associated with statins is above background risk
Bisphosphonates	All drugs in this class	Transient hypocalcaemia of newborn, low neonatal birth weight, skeletal abnormalities	Avoid during pregnancy	Caution— unknown if it enters breast milk	Caution using these medications in premenopausal women, since the drug remains present in bone for many years after use

Abbreviations: APS: antiphospholipid syndrome; CNS: central nervous system; LMWH: low-molecular weight heparin.

particularly at risk for spontaneous abortion, as well as worsening maternal renal activity during pregnancy.

The risk of pre-eclampsia in pregnant women with SLE varies amongst different studies. A nationwide study of all pregnancy-related hospitalizations between 2000 and 2003 revealed an incidence of pre-eclampsia in 22.5% of SLE pregnancies, which was three times higher than in the general population. The risk for pre-eclampsia is highest for women with active SLE nephritis at the time of pregnancy. Pregnant women with SLE have nearly twice the risk of undergoing Caesarean section delivery compared with pregnant women without SLE. The risk of intrauterine growth restriction is about three times higher than in healthy pregnant women without SLE. The risk of maternal death in pregnant women with SLE is up to 20 times higher than the general population. However, this is still a low absolute incidence, occurring in less than 0.5% of pregnancies.

There are other maternal risks for pregnant women with SLE. The risks of venous thromboembolism and stroke are up to 10 times higher in pregnant women with SLE compared with pregnant women without SLE. Women with antiphospholipid syndrome (APS) are at the highest risk of recurrent arterial thrombosis if they become pregnant. Pregnant women with SLE are also significantly more likely to have anaemia and thrombocytopenia compared with other pregnant women, and they are at increased risk for peripartum infections.

Neonatal lupus

A rare fetal complication is that of neonatal lupus. This is an autoimmune condition that occurs due to passive transfer of the maternal antibodies anti-SSA/Ro and anti-SSB/La across the placenta. Neonatal lupus occurs in 1–2% of pregnancies exposed to these maternal autoantibodies. It is not uncommon for neonatal lupus to be the initial presenting feature with subsequent development of maternal SLE, Sjogren's syndrome, or undifferentiated connective tissue disease. It primarily involves damage to the fetal heart including fibrosis of the cardiac conduction system, but there can also be hepatic or haematological involvement, and it can cause a rash after birth. Neonatal lupus can present with congenital heart block (CHB), which requires pacemaker placement in up to 60% of surviving babies within the first year of life. Rarely neonatal lupus with cardiac manifestations including CHB with cardiomyopathy can cause fetal death or premature death in surviving infants. The risk of poor outcome is increased if CHB is detected before 20 weeks gestation, if fetal heart rate is less than 50 beats per minute, if there is impaired fetal left ventricular dysfunction, or if there is hydrops fetalis (oedema of fetal compartments). The typical cutaneous manifestations of neonatal lupus are erythematous and scaling annular plaques, often involving the face and scalp. Typical haematological findings include pancytopenia or isolated anaemia, neutropenia, or thrombocytopenia. Hepatic involvement is usually seen as a transient transaminitis and/or conjugated hyperbilirubinaemia. In cases of neonatal lupus with predominately cutaneous, haematological, and/or hepatic manifestations, the outcome is usually benign as the condition resolves spontaneously and usually does not result in scarring of the skin.

Pregnant women at risk for neonatal lupus include those with a prior history of pregnancy complicated by neonatal lupus and those with SSA and SSB antibodies. There are no formal guidelines for antenatal screening for neonatal lupus, but it is generally recommended that these women should be screened with fetal heart rate monitoring between the 16th and 26th weeks gestation. If CHB is detected, fetal echocardiography should be obtained.

There is some evidence that treating the mother with hydroxychloroquine during pregnancy reduces the incidence of CHB. Therefore, this is a potential preventative treatment. In pregnancies with evidence of fetal conduction disease suggestive of neonatal lupus, fluorinated steroids can be administered to potentially decrease the risk of progressing to complete heart block. However, third degree congenital heart block has not been shown to be reversible despite fluorinated steroid use. Intravenous immune globulin (IVIG) and plasmapheresis have also been suggested as possible treatment options, but there is very limited evidence to support their use.

Exacerbation of SLE during pregnancy

There are mixed data regarding the risk of an SLE flare during pregnancy. In some patients, SLE activity is improved during pregnancy, while in other patients SLE activity is worsened during pregnancy. The risk of flare tends to depend on the pre-pregnancy SLE activity, whereas disease that is more quiescent pre-pregnancy is less likely to flare. When flares occur, they tend to be in the second or third trimester. Skin and joint symptoms are the most common manifestations of an SLE flare during pregnancy.

Distinguishing an SLE flare from normal pregnancy changes

As seen in Table 9.3, normal pregnancy is associated with several changes that could be confused with a lupus flare. A lesser degree of anaemia and thrombocytopenia is seen in normal pregnancy, related to increased plasma volume. Some proteinuria is normal in pregnancy, but greater than 2.6 g/L raises concern for abnormal proteinuria,

Table 9.3 Distinguishing a lupus flare from normal pregnancy changes			
		Normal pregnancy	Lupus flare
Laboratory features	Anaemia	Mild, Hb of 110+/– 2 g/L related to increased plasma volume	Can have more severe anaemia related to chronic inflammation or haemolytic anaemia
	Thrombocytopenia	Platelet count may decrease to low normal, usually not below 150×10^9/L	Can be decreased $< 100 \times 10^9$/L
	Complement levels	Usually increase	Either decrease or remain the same
	Proteinuria	Mild, up to 0.26 g in 24 hours	Can be elevated >0.5 g in 24 hours in lupus nephritis
	Creatinine	Lower than pre-pregnancy value, within normal range	May be increased in lupus nephritis
Clinical features	Cutaneous	Chloasma—'mask of pregnancy' with hyperpigmented patches involving the face	Malar rash—raised erythematous rash over cheeks/nose that spares nasolabial folds, discoid rash, vasculitis
	Musculoskeletal	Bland knee effusions	Inflammatory arthritis
	Cardiopulmonary	Dyspnoea and mild tachycardia	Pleurisy, pericarditis

such as due to lupus nephritis. Unlike with a lupus flare, in normal pregnancy the creatinine level will decrease. In pregnancy, complement levels should increase. Therefore, decreased or even stable complement levels during pregnancy raise concern for a possible SLE flare.

Distinguishing lupus nephritis from pre-eclampsia

A similar challenge involves distinguishing between SLE flares involving lupus nephritis and the pregnancy complication of pre-eclampsia. As seen in Table 9.4, there are several distinguishing features between the two disorders. Pre-eclampsia is defined by the presence of hypertension and proteinuria. It typically has onset after 20 weeks gestation. The exception is in SLE with severe APS, these women can develop early pre-eclampsia. Lupus nephritis can occur at any time and does not necessarily cause hypertension. There are several differentiating laboratory tests as well. In lupus nephritis, urinalysis will often reveal active urinary sediment including red and/or white cell casts. However, in pre-eclampsia the urinalysis will usually be bland with proteinuria. Women with SLE nephritis will often have positive anti-dsDNA antibodies, and the titres often rise with increased disease activity. Changes in autoantibodies are not seen with pre-eclampsia.

Contraception in women with SLE

The World Health Organization Medical Eligibility Criteria for Contraceptive Use guidelines recommend many contraceptive options for patients with SLE, including individuals using immunosuppressant medications. Barrier methods may be used as they help to reduce risk of transmission of infection, but they have the greatest risk of contraceptive failure resulting in unplanned pregnancy. The copper intrauterine device (IUD) is considered the safest option, and other options that are generally recommended for use include the levonorgestrel IUD, combined oral oestrogen/progesterone contraceptive pills, combined oestrogen/progesterone patch, progesterone-only pills, depot medroxyprogesterone acetate (DMPA) injections, and implantable oestrogen/progesterone devices. However, for women with SLE at higher risk for venous or arterial thrombosis, particularly including those with antiphospholipid syndrome (APS), caution must be taken in prescribing systemic hormonal methods of contraception,

Table 9.4 Distinguishing between lupus nephritis and pre-eclampsia

	Lupus nephritis	Pre-eclampsia
Timing of onset	Can occur at any time	Usually after 20 weeks of gestation
Associated hypertension	Sometimes present	Required for diagnosis, blood pressure >140/90 mmHg
Proteinuria	>5 g/L in 24 hour urine collection	>3 g/L in 24 hour urine collection
Urinalysis	Active urinary sediment	May be bland with proteinuria
Serum uric acid	Normal if no pre-existing renal damage	Will often be elevated
Urinary calcium excretion	Will be normal	Will often be reduced
Anti-dsDNA antibodies	Often present and titres usually rise with activity	Absent or unchanged from previous value

particularly those including oestrogens, as these medications could further increase the risk of thrombosis. Therefore, in APS and other patients with a history of thrombophilia, the copper IUD or the levonorgestrel IUD are the preferred methods of contraception. The progesterone-only pill and DMPA are alternative options in this case. If combined hormonal methods of contraception are chosen in patients with SLE, generally the lowest effective dose of oestrogen should be used, and 3rd and 4th generation progestins (eg, drospirenone) should be avoided due to increased risk for venous thromboembolism.

Safety and efficacy of pharmacotherapy for SLE during pregnancy and lactation

In pregnant patients with SLE, the choice of medications to treat SLE disease activity and other associated medical conditions should include a consideration of the maternal and fetal risks of these medications. It is important to weigh the potential risks of adverse effects of a medication against the risks of untreated maternal disease. The United States Federal Drug Administration (FDA) previously categorized medications for safety in pregnancy and lactation with the A, B, C, D, X categories. However, in June 2015, this categorization changed to the new Pregnancy and Lactation Labelling Rule (PLLR).

As seen in Table 9.1, some medications used to manage SLE disease activity are contraindicated in pregnancy whereas others are generally thought to be safe. Hydroxychloroquine is generally considered safe in pregnancy and there is increasing evidence that it may improve fetal outcomes, so there is no need to stop it before or during pregnancy. However, other medications including methotrexate, mycophenolate, cyclophosphamide, and leflunomide are contraindicated due to established risks of fetal harm. In addition to fetal risks, cyclophosphamide increases the risk of future infertility in women who are exposed. This risk may depend on the cumulative dose given, and lower dose regimens such as the Euro-Lupus regimen of cyclophosphamide may be associated with improved future fertility. Leflunomide causes multiple fetal anomalies in animal studies, and this medication remains present for up to two years after discontinuation of use. Standard practice is to document undetectable plasma levels of leflunomide prior to attempting conception. If unplanned pregnancy occurs, colestyramine washout should be performed with subsequent documentation of undetectable plasma levels. No increased risk of congenital abnormalities has been observed with this practice. For azathioprine, the majority of this drug is not converted to its active metabolite 6-mercaptopurine (6-MP) by the fetal liver. Therefore, the theoretical fetal risks are low. Recent studies have not found an increased risk of fetal anomalies with azathioprine. This medication is the safest current option for treatment of SLE nephritis or other severe disease during pregnancy, and women with SLE nephritis who are planning pregnancy should be switched to azathioprine six months before conception to ensure control of maternal disease on this agent. There are limited data on the newer agent belimumab, but several normal pregnancy outcomes have been recorded in cases of maternal exposure. This medication is likely to be safe in the first trimester when the monoclonal antibody cannot cross the placenta.

Other medications that are commonly used in patients with SLE can also have fetal effects and should be considered carefully during pregnancy, as seen in Table 9.4. The choice of anticoagulation for venous thromboembolism is strongly influenced by the risk of teratogenic effects with oral agents, and heparin and low molecular weight heparins (LMWH) are the recommended choices. Non-fluorinated glucocorticoids, such as prednisone and prednisolone, are metabolized by placental 11-β-hydrogenase into inactive form. Therefore, they do not reach fetal circulation in high concentrations and are the preferred corticosteroids for use in pregnancy. However, fluorinated steroids such as beclometasone and dexamethasone do reach fetal circulation and can have fetal effects, both intended and unintended.

Pharmacotherapy and fertility in men with SLE

In treating men with SLE, it is important to consider the effects of medications on male fertility. The disease-modifying anti-rheumatic drugs (DMARDs) methotrexate and sulfasalazine may reduce sperm count, which can cause temporary infertility in males. However, this is rare and usually reversible with discontinuation of the medication. It has been recommended that men should discontinue methotrexate at least three months prior to attempting conception due to the possible risk of teratogenicity, as drug levels can remain elevated in gonadal tissues, but there is little evidence for teratogenicity. Cyclophosphamide can also cause male infertility by reducing the quality and quantity of sperm, and these effects can be permanent. The risk of infertility increases with higher cumulative doses of this medication and men should be counselled regarding this risk of infertility.

Antiphospholipid antibody syndrome and pregnancy

Antiphospholipid antibody syndrome (APS) is commonly associated with SLE, and this syndrome has strong pregnancy implications. APS causes increased risk of pre-eclampsia and placental insufficiency. It also increases the risk for spontaneous abortion, up to three times higher than in women with SLE but without APS. This risk of abortion can be up to 90% without treatment, but can be reduced to less than 25% in women treated with LMWH and aspirin during pregnancy. Pregnancy loss can be the first indication that an individual has APS, and APS should be considered in women with multiple pregnancy losses or with premature delivery related to pre-eclampsia.

Cardiovascular disease in SLE

Premature cardiovascular disease in SLE

Mortality in SLE is bimodal, with an initial peak in mortality due to disease activity and infections, and a second peak in mortality that occurs with long-standing SLE mainly due to cardiovascular disease (CVD). SLE is associated with the development of premature CVD, and cardiovascular events occur at younger ages. The incidence of CVD is increased at least 7-fold overall in patients with SLE compared with the general population. In young patients, the incidence of CVD is over 10-fold greater when compared with their healthy peers, and women with SLE in their 30s or 40s are 50 times more likely to have a myocardial infarction.

Factors contributing to cardiovascular disease in SLE

The aetiology of the increased incidence of CVD in patients with SLE is multifactorial, related to both the inflammation and damage from SLE and an increase in traditional risk factors for CVD in those with SLE. Regarding these traditional risk factors, patients with SLE have more obesity, diabetes mellitus, hypertension, and hyperlipidaemia compared with the general population. This may be due in part to the prolonged and/or cumulative use of glucocorticoids. Patients with SLE are also more likely to be sedentary, which also adds to the increased CVD risk. However, even after accounting for these traditional risk factors, patients with SLE have a significantly increased risk for CVD.

Inflammation from SLE disease activity contributes to premature progression of atherosclerosis and can also cause CVD via thromboembolism related to a hyper-coagulable state, including coronary heart disease and cerebrovascular accidents. The progression of atherosclerosis in SLE is multifactorial. This is caused in part by endothelial cell dysfunction, increased monocyte activation at the endothelial wall, and reduced ability to repair vascular damage in patients with SLE. Another factor that may be contributing to premature atherosclerosis in SLE is pro-inflammatory high-density lipoprotein (HDL). During the acute phase response with active SLE disease activity, HDL can be converted from the usual anti-inflammatory state to a pro-inflammatory state. Therefore, elevated HDL in patients with SLE is not always protective against CVD. This adds to the difficulty in interpreting CVD risk for individual patients with SLE. While current models of CVD risk used for the general population do not adequately gauge the risk of CVD in SLE patients, there is no widely used risk model to predict CVD in this population.

Additional tools can be utilized in risk stratifying patients with SLE regarding the devel-opment of CVD. Measurements of carotid plaque and carotid intima-media thickness (CIMT) have been shown to correlate with the risk of CVD events in asymptomatic women with SLE. The quantification of coronary artery calcifications on CT scan has also been shown to correlate with risk of CVD events in the general population, and this has been extrapolated to patients with SLE. Therefore, these findings on imaging indicate the presence of subclinical atherosclerosis and can be considered in the overall risk assessment for CVD in patients with SLE. Patients with higher SLE damage accrual, as measured by the SLICC/ACR (Systemic Lupus International Collaborating Clinics/ American College of Rheumatology) damage index, and longer SLE disease duration tend to have increased quantities of carotid plaque and coronary artery calcifications.

Management strategies for preventing premature cardiovascular disease in SLE

An important strategy in reducing risk of CVD in SLE includes controlling SLE disease activity to reduce inflammation and progression of atherosclerosis. In addition to the beneficial effects on controlling SLE activity, the antimalarial medication hydroxychlo-roquine has been shown to have favourable effects on the metabolic profile, including fasting lipids, as well as on serum glucose control. This medication has also been associ-ated with less progression of carotid plaque in some studies. Another strategy involves minimizing glucocorticoids, as higher cumulative doses and longer duration of treat-ment with glucocorticoids increases the risk of diabetes, hyperlipidaemia, and CVD. Doses equal to or greater than 20 mg daily of oral prednisone can increase the risk of cardiovascular events by 5-fold.

Guidelines from the European League Against Rheumatism (EULAR) recommend screening patients with SLE for modifiable risk factors for CVD on at least an annual basis. As seen in Box 9.1, this includes screening blood pressure, BMI, smoking status, physical activity level, blood glucose, and serum lipids. Treating the underlying condi-tions that predispose patients to developing CVD is very important in patients with SLE. All patients should be encouraged to refrain from smoking and to engage in regular physical activity. In the treatment of hypertension, SLE has often been considered a cardiac disease risk equivalent, similar to diabetes. The 8th Joint National Committee (JNC 8) guidelines on the treatment of hypertension in adults, give no clear target blood pressure for patients with SLE. However, the goal blood pressure for people

> ### Box 9.1 Modifying risk factors for cardiovascular disease
>
> - Minimize glucocorticoids, both duration of treatment and cumulative dose
> - Screen for hypertension at least annually
> - Screen for obesity with regular weight measurement/BMI assessment
> - Assess smoking status at least annually and counsel regarding tobacco cessation
> - Assess physical activity level and counsel regarding regular physical activity
> - Screen for diabetes regularly with fasting blood glucose and/or haemoglobin A1c
> - Screen for hyperlipidaemia with regular fasting lipid panels
> - Consider obtaining measurements of CIMT, carotid plaque, and/or coronary artery calcium for further risk stratification
> - Treat with hydroxychloroquine if no contraindications or intolerance
> - Treat with daily low dose aspirin in cases of antiphospholipid antibody syndrome and other high risk patients
> - Consider statin therapy on individual basis
>
> BMI: body mass index; CIMT: carotid intima-media thickness.

under age 60 and for those with diabetes or chronic kidney disease (CKD) of all ages is less than or equal to 140/90 mmHg. Therefore, for patients with SLE, blood pressure goals should be at least this stringent, and there is evidence to suggest that a lower goal of 130/80 mmHg is beneficial in SLE, particularly with coexisting CKD and/or diabetes mellitus. These guidelines should be applied in the context of each individual patient, and individualized blood pressure goals may be appropriate. EULAR recommends the use of angiotensin converting enzyme inhibitors (ACEi) and angiotensin receptor blockers (ARBs) as first-line agents in treating hypertension in patients with SLE. Calcium-channel blockers are also acceptable alternatives, and they can be used particularly in patients with concomitant Raynaud's phenomenon. Beta-blockers should be avoided when possible to prevent worsening if Raynaud's symptoms are present.

Another mainstay of treatment to reduce CVD risk in the general population is the use of statins. The 2013 American College of Cardiology/American Heart Association (ACC/AHA) guidelines on the treatment of cholesterol in the general population for primary prevention of CVD, focus on treatment with statins for adults which depend on an individual's 10-year risk of CVD, rather than targeting particular goal cholesterol values; whereas prior recommendations focused on target low-density lipoprotein (LDL) levels. Previously, the target LDL goal was <2.50 mmol/L for patients with SLE. It is unclear how to apply the newer guidelines to patients with SLE at this time. The current ACC/AHA CVD risk calculator includes sex, age, race, total cholesterol, HDL cholesterol, systolic blood pressure, diabetes, and smoking status. However, this risk calculator underestimates the risk of CVD in patients with SLE. Additionally, the benefit of statins in patients with SLE is less clear than in the general population. There is limited longitudinal data regarding the use of statins and CVD outcomes in patients with SLE; smaller studies have shown an unclear benefit, suggesting that the treatment strategy of using statins to reduce future cardiovascular events may be less efficacious in patients with SLE. Therefore, the optimal use of statins in this population is not clearly established, and treatment decisions should be individualized for each patient.

There is some evidence to suggest the use of low dose aspirin (75 mg or 81 mg) daily for primary prevention of cardiovascular events in patients with SLE. In the absence of a contraindication, aspirin can be considered for all patients with SLE. However, it should particularly be considered for patients with a known history of CVD, or with hypertension, diabetes, hyperlipidaemia, or tobacco use.

Bone health in SLE

Women and men with SLE have a higher incidence of osteopenia and osteoporosis when compared with healthy peers. Up to 10–20% of premenopausal women with SLE have osteoporosis. This increased risk is largely due to the use of glucocorticoids, the use of other medications that promote bone loss, and higher rates of vitamin D deficiency in patients with SLE. Glucocorticoids are the most common cause of drug-induced osteoporosis. The long-term use of 7.5 mg or more of prednisone daily can cause adverse effects on bone mineral density. Several other medications that are commonly used by patients with SLE are also associated with an increased risk of bone mineral density loss. These include methotrexate, cyclophosphamide, ciclosporin, heparin, proton-pump inhibitors, and some antidepressants.

Prevention of osteoporosis in SLE

There are several recommended measures to reduce the risk of osteoporosis in patients with SLE, as seen in Box 9.2. One important strategy is to minimize the use of glucocorticoids. Steroid-sparing agents should be used whenever possible. Patients who will be taking glucocorticoids for durations greater than or equal to 3 months should be started on calcium and vitamin D supplementation. This should include 1200–1500 mg/day of calcium and 1000–2000 IU of vitamin D. These patients should also be screened for vitamin D deficiency and assessed for fall risk and for a history of fragility fractures. Particularly in older individuals, it is recommended to obtain a baseline height measurement and to assess for vertebral fracture in the setting of significant height loss. All patients with SLE on chronic glucocorticoids should also be counselled to engage in weight-bearing physical activities.

Screening for osteoporosis in SLE

Regarding screening for osteoporosis, the American College of Rheumatology recommends obtaining baseline bone mineral density (BMD) testing with a dual-energy X-ray

---

Box 9.2 Recommendations for reducing the risk of osteoporosis in patients with SLE taking chronic glucocorticoids

- Use the minimum effective dose of glucocorticoids and for the minimal necessary duration
- Screen for vitamin D deficiency annually
- Assess fall risk
- Obtain baseline height measurement
- Consider evaluation for vertebral fracture with X-ray if significant height loss
- Counsel patients to avoid excess alcohol use
- Counsel patients to avoid tobacco use
- Counsel patients to engage in regular weight-bearing exercises
- Supplement calcium and vitamin D (1200–1500 mg/day calcium and at least 1000–2000 IU/day of vitamin D)
- Obtain baseline bone mineral density measurement with DXA scan

absorptiometry (DXA) measurement in all patients who are taking long-term glucocorticoids (3 months or longer). However, there is no consensus on the frequency of bone mineral density testing, particularly for premenopausal women and men <50 years of age. The frequency of DXA testing should be individualized for each patient depending on the duration and cumulative dose of glucocorticoids, the use of other medications that increase fracture risk, age, other risk factors for fragility fracture, and the baseline BMD.

Treatment of osteoporosis in SLE

The approach to treatment of osteoporosis in patients with SLE depends on menopausal status, age, and sex. For premenopausal women and men under age 50, there is less evidence to suggest the use of prescription osteoporosis therapy, including bisphosphonates and the recombinant parathyroid hormone teriparatide. These treatments are generally reserved for patients in this category with history of fragility fracture, with very low bone mineral density and the need to continue with chronic glucocorticoid treatment, or with very low bone mineral density and the need for long-term heparin therapy. Bisphosphonates should be avoided in women of childbearing age as they can cause abnormal fetal skeletal development, even if conception occurs several years after maternal treatment with one of these agents. Teriparatide is not approved in pregnant or lactating women. Bisphosphonates pose additional risks to premenopausal women and younger men. These agents can lead to abnormal bone formation and increase the risk of complex fractures after five years of use. Therefore, they should generally be not taken long-term. If premenopausal women do require bisphosphonates, shorter-acting agents such as risedronate should be used. For postmenopausal women and for men over age 50, the risk of osteoporotic fracture should be assessed using the Fracture Risk Assessment Tool (FRAX). Low risk postmenopausal patients on >7.5 mg/day of glucocorticoids generally are recommended to start bisphosphonate therapy. Moderate and high-risk patients in this category generally qualify for pharmacologic treatment including bisphosphonates if they are on any maintenance dose of corticosteroids.

Prevention of infections in SLE

Patients with SLE are at increased risk for infectious complications. An important but often overlooked strategy in infection prevention is to ensure that these patients receive appropriate vaccinations. There are mixed data regarding the possible risk of an SLE flare after receiving immunizations, but the benefit generally outweighs this risk. Some patients with SLE have diminished protective antibody formation in response to vaccines. However, the majority of patients will have a successful immune response. When possible, patients with SLE should be vaccinated when SLE disease activity is low and before starting immunosuppressant therapy.

Recommended vaccinations in SLE

Inactivated/killed vaccines are generally safe in patients who are receiving immunosuppressant medications. Attenuated live vaccines are contraindicated in patients on moderate immunosuppression regimens that are equivalent to >20 mg per day of prednisone, <0.4 mg/kg/week of methotrexate, or <3 mg/kg of azathioprine daily, due to the risk of disseminated infection. Live attenuated vaccines including measles mumps and rubella (MMR) and the herpes zoster vaccine may be safe in patients with SLE who are only mildly immunosuppressed.

The inactivated vaccines for influenza virus, pneumococcal pneumonia, tetanus toxoid, and human papilloma virus are all recommended for patients with SLE. It is strongly recommended that patients with SLE should receive yearly influenza vaccines, as they are at increased risk for complications of influenza virus. Pneumococcal vaccinations with killed, conjugated vaccines are also recommended by EULAR in patients with SLE, as SLE patients are at higher risk of developing pneumococcal pulmonary infections than the general population. In the United States of America, the Advisory Committee on Immunization Practices (ACIP) recommends the pneumococcal polysaccharide vaccine (PCV13) followed by the 23-valent polysaccharide vaccine (PPSV23). Patients with SLE should receive the tetanus toxoid vaccine as per the same schedule as the general population. The inactivated human papilloma virus vaccine is also recommended. Women with SLE have a higher incidence of HPV infection and have reduced viral clearance, which emphasizes the importance of vaccinating this population against HPV.

Additional strategies to prevent infections in SLE

Patients with SLE should be screened for several common bacterial and viral infections. Those with risk factors and those preparing to start immunosuppressive therapy should be screened for tuberculosis, hepatitis C virus, hepatitis B virus, and human immunodeficiency virus (HIV). Antimicrobial prophylaxis should also be given in certain circumstances. Patients with SLE on high levels of immunosuppression and with lymphopenia, particularly with lymphocyte counts under $1 \times 10^9/L$, are at risk for *Pneumocystis jirovecii* pneumonia (PJP). Prophylactic treatment with trimethoprim-sulfamethoxazole (co-trimoxazole) or other agents against PJP should be considered on an individual basis since there are no clear guidelines for when to initiate this treatment and some SLE patients do not tolerate sulfonamides. Another risk for infectious complications is that patients with SLE who are treated with immunosuppressants can develop secondary immunodeficiencies. Patients with SLE who develop secondary hypogammaglobulinaemia or specific antibody deficiency along with recurrent infectious can be given immunoglobulin replacement with intravenous immune globulin (IVIG).

Malignancy in SLE

An increased incidence of malignancy is seen in patients with SLE. The individual risk is increased by 15% compared to the general population. These patients have a unique risk profile for certain malignancies. This is likely to be related to altered immune function as well as to treatment with cytotoxic medications. Given the increased risk for malignancies, routine cancer screening is an important part of treating patients with SLE.

Cancer risk in SLE

There is an increased risk of non-Hodgkin's lymphoma in SLE patients of three times that of the general population. Most commonly, this is diffuse, large B-cell lymphoma. Patients with SLE also have an increased risk of cervical cancer, which may be related to the reduced ability to clear the human papilloma virus (HPV). There is also an increased incidence of lung and possibly liver cancer in individuals with SLE compared to the general population. Large population studies have shown possibly decreased incidences of breast and endometrial cancer in women with SLE. However, some smaller studies have shown higher rates of these malignancies in SLE patients. The variable risk for these cancers may be related to differences in ethnic backgrounds.

Cancer screening in SLE

There are no published guidelines regarding unique cancer screening in SLE patients. Patients with SLE should generally receive at least the recommended age-appropriate cancer screening for the general population. However, SLE patients generally have much lower rates of adherence to these screening guidelines. In addition to standard screening, some experts recommend intensified cervical cancer screening with yearly Papanicolaou testing, but there are no clinical trials to support this. There is currently no evidence to suggest routine screening for additional malignancies such as lung cancer in patients with SLE, but patients should be advised to quit smoking as tobacco use increases the risk of lung cancer more in lupus patients than in the general population.

Further reading

Andreoli L, Fredi M, Nalli C, et al. Pregnancy implications for systemic lupus erythematosus and the antiphospholipid syndrome. *J Autoimmun* 2012;38:197–208.

Bertsias G, Ioannidis JPM, Boletis J, et al. EULAR recommendations for the management of systemic lupus erythematosus. Report of a Task Force of the EULAR Standing Committee for International Clinical Studies Including Therapeutics. *Ann Rheum Dis* 2008;67:195–205.

Bichile T, Petri M. Prevention and management of co-morbidities in SLE. *Presse Medicale* 2014;43:e187–95.

Cloutier BT, Clarke AE, Ramsey-Goldman R, Gordon C, Hansen JE, Bernatsky S. Systemic lupus erythematosus and malignancies: a review article. *Rheum Dis Clin North Am* 2014;40:497–506.

Flint J, Panchal S, Hurrell A, et al. BSR and BHPR guideline on prescribing drugs in pregnancy and breastfeeding. Part I: standard and biologic disease modifying anti-rheumatic drugs and corticosteroids. Pre-press, available at http://www.rheumatology.org.uk/includes/documents/cm_docs/2015/f/full_guideline_part_i.pdf (Accessed 9 Sept 2015).

Grossman JM, et al., American College of Rheumatology 2010 recommendations for the prevention and treatment of glucocorticoid-induced osteoporosis. *Arthritis Care Res* 2010;62:1515–26.

Lin P, Bonaminio P, Ramsey-Goldman R. Chapter 14: Pregnancy and rheumatic disease. In Imboden JB, Hellmann DB, Stone JH. *Current rheumatology diagnosis and treatment.* 2nd Ed. New York, USA, McGraw-Hill Companies, Inc., 2007:146–59.

Østensen M, Andreoli L, Brucato A, et al. State of the art: Reproduction and pregnancy in rheumatic diseases. *Autoimmun Rev* 2015:14;376–386.

Peart E, Clowse MEB. Systemic lupus erythematosus and pregnancy outcomes: an update and review of the literature. *Curr Opin Rheumatol* 2014;26:118–23.

Shoback D. Chapter 57: Osteoporosis and glucocorticoid-induced osteoporosis. In Imboden JB, Hellmann DB, Stone JH. *Current rheumatology diagnosis and treatment.* 2nd Ed. New York, USA, McGaw Hill Companies Inc., 2007.

Skaggs B, Hahn B, McMahon M. Accelerated atherosclerosis in patients with SLE-mechanisms and management. *Nat Rev Rheumatol* 2012;8:214–23.

Soh MC, Nelson-Piercy C. High-risk pregnancy and the rheumatologist. *Rheumatology* 2015;54:572–87.

van Assen S, Agmon-Levin N, Elkayam O, et al. EULAR recommendations for vaccination in adult patients with autoimmune inflammatory rheumatic diseases. *Ann Rheum Dis* 2011;70:414–22.

Index

Tables, figures, and boxes are indicated by an italic *t*, *f*, and *b* following the page number.

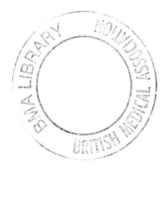